Chair Exercises for Seniors

Stay Strong and Balanced with 7 Daily Low-Impact Routines; Reduce Pain, Prevent Falls, and Improve Mobility for a Healthier, More Independent Lifestyle

Luke Adams

Inkwell Foundry

Contents

Introduction

> Aging is not lost youth but a new stage of opportunity and strength.
>
> Betty Friedan

I believe wholeheartedly in this statement. Getting older is a privilege that comes with a multitude of opportunities to grow mentally, physically, and spiritually.

How we choose to handle and navigate this chapter of life will set the course for the remaining years. I choose to go into this phase as strongly as I can within all facets of my life.

Like you, I believed that my best years were behind me. I felt that my youth was slowly slipping away and that my goals and desires had already passed me by. I was over at my mother's assisted living facility, where I met one of the most energetic, upbeat, and positive people I have ever encountered. Her name was Harriet and she was 87 years old.

Harriet was passionate about her life, and she spoke about her hobbies and interests with great enthusiasm. Harriet explained that most of her newfound interests were found later in life—her later years had allowed her to explore and discover new interests. Her energy and passion was infectious, especially for my mother.

After seeing how enthusiastic my mother had become about her newfound interest in the piano, I realized that this period of life could bring about many new and exciting things.

I left feeling inspired and decided to start writing again—a practice I had put off for years. I had always wanted to write a book, and since my children were grown, my career was stable, and I had the extra time, so I decided to go for it. And so, this book was born.

Aging is a complex and confusing time to navigate, but it is not the time to give up on your dreams. Yes, we are getting older each year, but this is not the time to sit back and let it overcome us.

I understand that the physical changes of increasing age can also negatively affect your mental health, resulting in discouragement seeping into your day-to-day activities. These feelings are normal. Issues such as mobility impairment may hinder your ability to move freely, thus holding you back from the activities you once enjoyed or discouraging you from pursuing. Your social life may have suffered and you may fear the loss of your independence. Or you may inadvertently begin to isolate yourself from your community because you have these underlying fears and a loss of faith in your physical capabilities.

According to Freiberger et al. (2020), we will be at a greater risk of falling once we begin to have balance and mobility issues. Research has shown that approximately 27% of adults aged 45–79 in the United States have taken a fall in the past year or so; of that number, 11% resulted in a serious injury. All these negative thoughts may weigh heavily on your mind these days and may be holding you back.

I am going to present one solution to you: exercise. Lack of physical activity, strength, balance impairment, weight issues, and chronic disease are all risk factors for mobility problems, and exercise is one of the best-recommended tools to combat this.

If you can intentionally keep active with both exercise and by moving more throughout your day, you can maintain or increase your strength, flexibility, balance, and endurance (Freiberger et al., 2020).

I won't deny that the physical changes we may be experiencing may lead us to have more difficulty in pursuing particular goals, but we do have the tools to counteract them. With the proper knowledge and guidance, we can develop and partake in an exercise routine that can provide us with an outlet and solution to adapt and overcome these challenges, enabling us to continue living fulfilling lives.

As we go through this journey together, I want us to focus on what we can do now rather than what we can no longer do. This mindset can make a world of difference.

I want to tell you about Joan. Joan is well known in the fitness industry, and you may have seen her on social media as @trainwithjoan. Joan decided when she was 70 years old that she needed to get healthy and make exercise a priority in life. She started an exercise routine, changed her diet, and prioritized her health. Exercise and diet significantly improved her life (MacDonald, n.d.).

In five short years, Joan went from being overweight, suffering from mobility issues, having multiple medical conditions, and taking many medications to treat her symptoms. She changed her life by becoming strong, confident, capable, and living an enriching lifestyle. She is proof, among other inspiring stories, that it is never too late to start.

You could, should, and will be doing this for yourself. It is your gift to both yourself and your future self. By the end of this book, I aim to have you moving with a confidence that will permeate into all the other areas of your life.

It will be hard work at times, but I promise it is worth it, and the results will always be satisfying. I look forward to helping you reduce pain, prevent falls, and improve your strength and mobility, thereby improving your overall quality of life.

When I began in this industry, I desired to write and help as many older adults as possible to have the strength and confidence to enjoy and pursue their passions, and now I am going for it. Please take my advice and go for yours! Whatever your reason for the change, let's do this together and begin today!

Stay In Sync With Your Body—The Changes

> Physical fitness is not only one of the most important keys to a healthy body, it is the basis of dynamic and creative intellectual activity.
>
> John F. Kennedy

With the advances in modern medicine, we are all living a lot longer than before. However, are we living in our healthiest state during those added years? Some of us may be, but we all have room to improve our lives.

I always think about lifespan versus health span. Lifespan is how long you live. Your health span is how long you live a healthy, vibrant life. Our goal is to get our health span to equal our lifespan. Researchers conducted an interesting study that looked at the Blue Zones of the world: areas where the populations live long and vibrant lives well into their later years.

Blue Zones are Okinawa, Japan; Sardinia, Italy; Nicoya, Costa Rica; Ikaria, Greece; and Loma Linda, California (Blue Zones, 2015). The people here have integrated certain practices and behaviors that have resulted in communities known for longevity, vitality, and wholesome quality of life. One of the most common practices of those living within these Blue Zones is regularly exercising and engaging in physical activity daily. They also sleep well, have a sense of community, and are social—all other aspects of life that greatly benefit from exercise.

This community routine has resulted in a gentle and manageable aging process. These Blue Zone communities have far fewer issues regarding certain aspects of growing older than other communities found elsewhere. Listed below are some of the expected changes that happen as we age.

Mobility

As we age, we become less capable of specific daily tasks. We lose muscle, our balance changes, and our joints may stiffen. This all results in decreased ease with which we get around and perform tasks. Please do not let a preventable fall occur before realizing you may have mobility issues. Here are some questions to ask yourself regarding your mobility.

Are you noticing that you can't walk or stand for as long as you used to? Or are you having difficulty getting up and down when you sit? These warning signs may not be a lack of fitness but rather a decline in mobility. Is your balance off or dexterity impaired? Other warning signs include dizziness or difficulty climbing stairs or stepping over objects. If you are finding it difficult to climb up ten steps, walk a quarter of a mile, or have had to modify specific tasks because of your physical condition, then you should seek advice from your healthcare provider (SonderCare, n.d.).

Along with general aging, there are other contributing factors to the decline in mobility.

Musculoskeletal System

As we age, we begin to lose muscle mass and bone density. Our bones become more fragile, and we are at greater risk of fractures should we fall. Osteoporosis is the medical terminology for significant bone loss. The fear of brittle bones can make us wary of activity, so we tend to avoid it; however, this common mistake leads to even more bone loss. It is a continuous cycle that exercise can correct.

Our muscles may become less flexible, and we risk losing endurance and strength, affecting our coordination, balance, and stability. Sarcopenia is the breakdown of muscle mass, resulting in a loss of strength.

Mayo Clinic (2020) recommends weight training or weight-bearing exercises to keep our bones strong and maintain muscle mass. Building and maintaining strength should be a priority as we age to ensure that our bodies can continue to keep up with the demanding tasks that life has for us. The more we strengthen the muscles around our bones, the more we protect and strengthen the bone structure.

We should also maintain appropriate calcium and vitamin D intake to keep our musculoskeletal system healthy.

Hearing and Sight

As we age, we experience changes in our vision and hearing which can play a role in our mobility as we may need help to move around as freely as we once did.

Visit your healthcare provider and get tested to determine whether you need glasses or a hearing aid. These simple healthcare accessories can restore confidence and independence.

Along with the development of cataracts, you may become sensitive to light and glare. Your hearing may suffer, and you could find it challenging to follow conversations or hear high frequencies.

Keep up with your medical checkups and see your optometrist and audiologist as often as you need. Preventative measures such as wearing a sun hat and using earplugs can also help reduce the risk of damage.

Neuromuscular Disorders

Neuromuscular disorders can affect our voluntary movement patterns as they tend to attack the nerves that control your nerves' automatic processes (May, 2020). Our legs are commonly negatively affected by neuromuscular disorders such as multiple sclerosis (MS) and muscular dystrophy.

Along with exercise, you may need additional aids to help you move about confidently.

The good news is that there are several things you can do to limit your decline in mobility that is associated with aging. It is most certainly not inevitable. Simple practices such as exercising, maintaining a healthy lifestyle, monitoring your weight, stopping smoking, and limiting your alcohol intake will help decrease your chances of losing mobility.

Pain

As we age, we may experience more aches and pains as we do our daily tasks. Chronic pain can be onset by various diseases such as arthritis, osteoporosis, diabetes, or neuromuscular and cardiovascular disease (Robeck, 2012).

Unfortunately, the onset of pain as we get older does not just hinder us physically but also has effects on our sleep and stress levels. Over time, frequent pain stress can cause or add to symptoms of depression and anxiety.

According to Dagnino & Campos (2022), our responses and our body's ability to manage and deal with pain change as we age. Our pain threshold may decrease as we age, and our bodies may experience an incline in painful sensations and a decrease in pain tolerance. Pain provides a warning system for our bodies: It tells us to avoid whatever we are doing as it is causing us discomfort and could be harmful. When the functionality of this warning system is constantly triggered, we are more likely to get injured as a result.

The pain cycle can create many limitations for us, but there are certain things we can do to prevent this from hindering our lives. We don't want chronic pain to take away our joy and independence or change our approach to the activities we currently do or want to do. We commonly become more sedentary due to pain issues, but this tactic will continue the pain cycle.

Understanding that our pain tolerance and triggers are not just a long and bumpy deteriorating road is essential. We can reset and train our pain system to work as initially intended. Decoupling our fear of pain and learning to understand what pain signals are trying to tell us goes a long way toward improving our relationship with our pain system response. The primary tool is gentle exercise with gradually increasing intensity over time. We need to keep moving, and we need to get and stay strong.

I am not asking you to push through any pain or injury—you should always work within your limits and consult your healthcare provider at the onset of any new or progressive pain.

When having a challenging day with pain, turning to making art or being around others, particularly family, pets, and animals, can reduce pain. Other non-pharmaceutical routes include cognitive behavioral therapy, progressive relaxation, mindfulness meditation, and pain neuroscience education (Dagnino & Campos, 2022). The one solution that I was particularly interested in was exercise. I urge you to keep moving, maintaining, and building your strength, especially if it becomes a struggle. Your body will thank you as you work to build a better relationship with your pain/discomfort awareness system.

Arthritis

Arthritis occurs when your joints become inflamed. It is a degenerative disease found more commonly in adults over 60 (The Most Common Causes of Limited Mobility in Seniors, n.d.). The disease can be painful and causes the joints to lock up and become stiff.

Arthritis is managed with medication and with physical therapy. Gentle exercise is one of the best tools to help ease the symptoms.

Cardiovascular System

The term cardiovascular relates to the heart, veins, and arteries. Issues with the heart and vascular structure can make circulating blood around the body challenging. Our blood vessels begin to harden and may stiffen, making our hearts work harder to pump blood through our bodies. Consequently, our resting heart rate will stay the same and not increase during activities. The heart working harder results in higher bouts of fatigue that occur more often and for extended periods. Everyday tasks and movements become exhausting and difficult. Over time, untreated vascular issues may trigger high blood pressure and other cardiovascular-related illnesses.

By managing your blood pressure and cholesterol levels via medication or exercise, you can lessen the risk of heart disease, improve circulation and strengthen your heart and vascular system. Other ways to control our risks and symptoms are eating healthy, managing stress, and getting enough sleep (Mayo Clinic, 2020).

The Risk of Falls

Falls are the leading cause of injury and death amongst the 65+ population, with statistics from the CDC (2020) showing that an older adult falls every second in the United States alone. Out of every five falls, one will result in a head injury or broken bones. Several factors contribute to falling, such as:

- advanced age
- fear of falling
- previous falls
- poor vision or hearing problems
- gait or balance problems
- muscle weakness
- postural hypotension
- chronic conditions, including arthritis, stroke, incontinence, diabetes, Parkinson's, and dementia

Those are some worrying figures, but you do not need to become one of those statistics. We can set ourselves up to ensure we are stable on our feet with simple things like focusing on balance exercises and becoming more aware of our surroundings and limitations. Exercise will keep our lower limbs strong, improve reaction time, and keep us more in tune with our bodies and how they move and change.

The first way to start is to ensure we are on top of our health. Visit your optometrist at least once a year to have your eyes assessed. Having your feet and gait checked out by a podiatrist would also be beneficial—gait often changes as we age and can contribute to your potential fall risk. As we get older, our hearing also changes, and according to the National Council On Aging (2023), you are three times more likely to fall should you have mild hearing loss.

The majority of falls take place in the home. Take a look at your surroundings, assess your living space, and design your home to be more user-friendly. Remove anything that may be a tripping hazard, improve lighting, and place objects used often in places that are easy to access. Remove rugs and be mindful of surfaces that may be slippery.

Balance and Coordination Issues

The good news is that, even though you may be experiencing a decline in balance and coordination, you can practice and maintain these skills. Exercise will help you get stronger by working your muscles and developing the skills needed to keep you stable while on your feet.

If your balance problems seem too severe, speak to your healthcare provider, as you may be suffering from an ear-related imbalance. They can inform you if it is a general issue or something tied to a peripheral vestibular dysfunction (The Most Common Causes of Limited Mobility in Seniors, n.d.).

Other Changes

Digestive System

As we age, we may experience more incidences of constipation due to the changes that are taking place in our large intestines. Along with these structural changes, lack of exercise, insufficient hydration, lack of fiber, and certain medications can also contribute to this issue.

Some advice from the Mayo Clinic (2020) is to listen to your body when it comes to bowel movements and not hold in a bowel movement for too long. Pay attention to your fiber intake, adjust your diet to include more fiber-rich foods, and exercise often.

Urinary System

As we age, our bladder loses elasticity which can result in us needing to urinate more frequently. Your bladder and pelvic floor muscles may also weaken, leading to incontinence and the inability to empty your bladder fully.

To keep your urinary system healthy, go to the toilet frequently and avoid getting a full bladder. Do core exercises to keep your muscles strong and functional and avoid bladder irritants. It is also important to maintain a healthy weight and refrain from smoking.

Cognitive Function

Memory and thinking skills may decline the older we get. Simple things such as multitasking or remembering names or words may become more strenuous to retain and grasp. We naturally lose cells as we age, and our brain cells are no different. Along with losing cells, we lose our memory, our reflexes slow, and we find ourselves distracted easier.

Alzheimer's disease, Parkinson's disease, and dementia are three of the primary cognitive disorders that could affect our mobility. These diseases make it difficult to control our bodies, thus making simple, everyday tasks difficult to manage.

The key is to stay mentally, physically, and socially active. Take up a new hobby, join classes, read, learn to play an instrument, or even play word games. Keep an active social life and integrate into a community. Social interaction has been known to ward off depression and stress and aid your mental health. Visit your friends, join a local community center or volunteer. It is common to isolate ourselves as we age, which has far-reaching adverse consequences on our mental health.

In most cases, cognitive decline is relatively mild and does not drastically affect the day-to-day functioning of most people (American Psychological Association, 2021). You are also more likely to notice changes in short-term memory as opposed to long-term memory, and although it may take longer, you will also be able to learn new things as you get older.

More importantly, it has been shown that as we age, we tend to become more at peace with life. We retain our optimism and look forward to the upcoming years.

Weight Issues

Changes in our metabolism can create a calorie imbalance, and we eat more food than we need, resulting in weight gain. We also tend to reduce the amount of activity we do as we age. Monitoring our food intake and ensuring we eat healthily and stay active will help manage our weight.

Being overweight can put extra stress on your joints, bones, and muscles, causing difficulties when moving. Obesity also increases your risk of developing other diseases, such as osteoarthritis and diabetes, which contribute to decreased mobility. Exercise and a good nutrition plan can help you maintain your weight as your metabolism and activity levels change as you get older.

It is also important to remember that you are an individual and, depending on your current health, your experiences with weight management could be very different from someone else. This list of changes may seem overwhelming, but I assure you it's not all doom and gloom. You have begun the journey to change what it means to age by focusing on your physical well-being. Many of the conditions listed above can be managed with an effective exercise program, and you have one in your hands.

Other practices that can help the aging process:
- Engage in preventive health behaviors.
- Educate yourself on the aging process.
- Be your personal health advocate.
- Look after your mental health.

Exercise Is the Answer

There may be things that you believe will prevent you from exercising or that make you wary of exercise: mobility issues, flexibility limitations, injuries, poor balance or posture, lack of experience, or just general age. If anything, those reasons should be your reason to turn to exercise.

It is never too late, and you are certainly young enough to begin working out for your health. I cannot highlight the benefits enough.

Benefits of Exercise

By using a combination of strength training, aerobic capacity training, and training that focuses on flexibility and balance, you can substantially alter the progression of your aging process. Exercise has many other benefits for everyone, regardless of age, along with improved physical capabilities, mental wellness, and emotional regulation.

Improves Health

The first and most obvious benefit is that exercise improves health across the board.

An overly sedentary lifestyle can increase your risk of developing cardiovascular disease, chronic illnesses, certain cancers, and obesity. Exercise can help lessen your risk of developing these diseases by keeping your immune system strong and functioning optimally.

If you already suffer from obesity, cardiovascular disease, chronic illness, or cancer, exercise can help you manage your symptoms. If you suffer from mental health conditions, exercise has also been shown to be effective in managing these issues as well.

Physical activity is one of the single most important things you can do to improve your longevity.

Protects Bones

Bone is living tissue that is continually being broken down and regrown. This natural process is called bone resorption (John Hopkins

Medicine, n.d.). Exercise builds muscle and helps our bones rejuvenate cells, making them denser and more robust.

The older we get, the less dense our bones become, and the more likely our risk of obtaining fractures or severe breaks should we fall. Exercise stimulates our bones to stay strong and can even strengthen them more if performed often and well.

Prevents Falls

Building strength can make you stronger and more confident on your feet. Not only can it help you to prevent falling by making sure you are stable, but it can also be the deciding factor in the severity of the injury.

If you have been exercising and maintaining your strength, you will likely have a less severe fall due to your strength and general fitness. In addition, your recovery may be more manageable.

Incorporate balance training in your regime and maintain that confidence on your feet. Often, our fear of falling holds us back from many activities we may want to participate in, exercise being one of them.

Manages Pain

Arthritis is a painful disease that affects the joints and is a common ailment in our aging community. You may wonder how exercise can help a disease that causes pain whenever you move. Still, it has been shown that arthritis-friendly exercises can have a positive effect on the intensity of the pain you may experience.

Exercise supports, maintains, and builds the muscles around the joints, keeping them protected and taking the pressure off the joint.

Exercise also reduces inflammation and aids in lubricating the joints for easier movement (National Council of Aging, n.d.).

Manages Body Weight

Specific changes to our metabolism and hormones can make it easier to gain and more challenging to lose weight. Certain medications can have this effect as well.

Exercise and good nutrition can help manage potential weight gain and help you lose weight should your health require it. Additionally, muscle increases metabolism, so maintaining and building muscle can positively affect your metabolic function.

Promotes Good Sleep

Sleep is vital for essential bodily functions and health. Keeping active can help you fall asleep and have better quality sleep. The physical exertion of exercise can tire you out, and the change in body temperature as you work out will help your body downregulate and relax.

It is also interesting to note that exercise will give you more energy for the day ahead. It also improves cognitive function and focus.

Improves Mental Health

Exercise makes us feel good due to the release of endorphins.

As we age, we may experience a dip in mood and, in some extreme instances, anxiety and depression. It is normal to feel emotional, considering all the changes we are going through; however, exercise can help alleviate this. Endorphins are chemicals the body creates that improve mood and create feelings of calmness and happiness. They can also help with symptoms of anxiety and stress.

Exercising is also an excellent way to socialize, whether you join an exercise group, attend a yoga class, or meet others while out taking a walk. The community aspect it creates can be very beneficial to your mental health.

If you are exercising and socializing and notice a very prominent dip in your mood that you cannot shake, please chat with your healthcare provider. Although feeling down can be a normal occurrence, depression and very intense periods of sadness may need professional help.

Myths About Exercising as an Older Adult

Now you know the benefits of exercise and its positive effects on your life. However, there may still be some hesitation regarding some information that is out there.

I want to touch on some of the myths that may be holding you back and have you second-guessing your decision. Consider this another nudge towards the path of health and fitness.

It Is Too Late for Me

Absolutely not! It is the perfect time to start, as it is never too late to begin working on your health again. Small changes now will have lasting impacts in the future.

I have written this book to give you a starting point and an easy-to-follow routine that you can implement into your life and begin to feel and see the results in just weeks.

Regardless of whether you have never been active before or have taken years off of activity, exercise will bring you only positive results in most areas of your life.

Do not give up on yourself. It is never too late to start investing in your well-being, as there is no age limit for good health. We are embarking on this journey for longevity to improve the years of our lives that we still have to live. The sooner we start to work on our fitness, the longer we maintain it and the more we can do with our lives.

I Am No Longer Athletic

It serves no positive purpose to compare yourself to past versions of yourself. You may have been very impressive on a basketball field or a very fit long-distance runner, but life has changed, and you and your capabilities have changed along with it.

There are many ways that you can look at and appreciate your current fitness status; the mere fact that you have a body that is capable of activity is one way to celebrate yourself.

Set some goals you want to accomplish and work towards them when you begin this journey. The milestones you set can help you realize how far you have come and motivate you to go even further than you may think possible.

My Health Issues Will Hold Me Back

Take the time to investigate whether this holds true by sitting down with your healthcare provider. Your doctor will likely encourage you to proceed with the exercise training program as it positively affects most symptoms and diseases.

Exercise is a proven tool to manage many conditions, such as diabetes and high blood pressure; as previously mentioned, it also helps manage pain.

I Am Disabled

Many programs can cater to those who may be disabled, ranging from chair exercises to weight lifting. The key is to be able to modify certain movements to cater to your needs.

It is most certainly worth investigating the options.

If you have any of the above concerns, raise them at your next health-care appointment. Knowing your medical history, your doctor can advise you on the steps to begin exercising.

Why Chair Exercises?

> You are never too old to set another goal or to dream a new dream.
>
> C.S. Lewis

I firmly believe that age does not limit us, and we are not too old to create a better life as we embark on the following chapters of our journey.

It may seem challenging or daunting, but at the end of the day, your health is worth it. Don't let your mind hold you back from the things you are capable of, even if it may be overwhelming. Life is constantly in motion, and pursuing your passions and dreams is never too late.

Your goal is to maintain quality of life and to continue on a path of longevity. We are going to use exercise to accomplish this—specifically, chair exercises.

So as we approach this form of exercise, look at it with curiosity and excitement. This is a great way to combat fear or apprehension before starting a new exercise regime. Taking small steps is the way to do it, so for now, we will learn what you will be doing so that you have the knowledge and confidence behind your actions.

What Are Chair Exercises?

As the name implies, chair exercises utilize a chair as the main component of the fitness routine. These can be done by those who have limited mobility, injuries, physical limitations, or diseases such as arthritis, Parkinson's, or MS. They can also be done by office workers who spend most of their day sitting and would like to either add more movement to their days or break up the frequent periods of inactivity.

These exercises are great for adding low-impact activity to one's day and do not require much extra effort to set up. In addition, they can be done without any special equipment apart from a suitable chair, if needed.

Chair exercises are also not only limited to seated movements, but often some exercises are performed using the chair as a prop to balance or offer support to the movements. The great thing about chair exercises is that they can be scaled and adapted to be more difficult or easier, depending on your fitness level.

Benefits of Chair Exercises

Chair exercises offer a safe, low-impact, and easily accessible way to work out while still providing the mental and physical benefits that come with conventional exercise programs.

Improves Posture

Years spent sitting and a general shift towards more sedentary behavior have resulted in numerous health problems, including poor posture. The more time we spend sitting, the more strain our joints and muscles experience. Biological design intended humans to move and to move often.

Due to the inactivity, our joints and muscles may begin to stiffen, and the shift in posture may become permanent if not tended to and can lead to pain and discomfort. Muscles, such as the glutes and core, may begin to weaken, and the cycle will continue as your posture worsens and your body struggles to manage the load (Care Link, 2021).

Specific chair exercises such as belly breathing and basic shoulder rolls can help improve your posture.

Increases Coordination

Coordination and balance can decrease as we age, so we must be mindful to continue building and maintaining hand-eye coordination. Repetitive exercises such as seated rotations can build muscle memory and coordination.

Alleviates Pain

Exercise releases endorphins to help inflammation, and movement keeps joints lubricated and muscles strong. Strong muscles mean less pressure on tendons and muscles which, in turn, results in less pain.

The advice to move more is recommended because movement provides our body pain relief; as I mentioned before, we were not designed to spend hours sitting. Our sedentary lifestyle is not suited for our bodies.

Chair exercises and seated stretches can be beneficial in alleviating pain. Remember never to push yourself into pain; consult a healthcare provider if you experience new pain and discomfort.

Improves Cardiovascular Health and Blood Circulation

Chair exercises will elevate your heart rate, which benefits your heart health. The movement will help pump blood and oxygen around your body and increase blood circulation. As we age, we often experience poor circulation, which can result in numbness in our limbs, digestive issues, and even a decline in energy levels (Scalena, 2021).

Disease Prevention

Exercise lowers the risk of high cholesterol, high blood pressure, and stress. These increase your risk of developing certain diseases such as heart attacks and strokes (Hanna & Norman, n.d.).

Manages Weight

Chair exercises can help you burn calories which will help you maintain your weight. Weight gain is a potential as we age due to the changes in our metabolism and activity levels. Chair exercises will also help you maintain muscle mass, thus keeping your metabolism functioning optimally.

Enhances Memory and Cognitive Function

According to research, just six months of regular exercise can boost memory and cognitive function, thus improving thinking and memory skills. Regular exercise has also been shown to increase blood and oxygen to the brain and help build more cells and neural pathways (Scalena, 2021).

Improves Mental Health

Endorphins are considered feel-good hormones and are released when we exercise. Exercise has been shown to reduce stress and anxiety and relieve symptoms of depression. It also has a positive impact on your sleep, which aids in mental clarity and health.

Safety Tips When Beginning

Before we delve into the nuances of how to begin exercising safely, the first thing you should always do before embarking on any health and fitness regime is to consult with your health and fitness provider.

Usually, a health provider will either know your pre-existing medical and fitness history or screen you to determine your current status. Your doctor can provide important background information that may influence your training program.

It is important to keep your doctor informed throughout this process as well. Keep them updated with your routines and any other health changes you may be experiencing as you continue to get fitter and stronger.

Questions to Ask Your Doctor

- What type of exercises should I be focusing on?
- Are there any activities or exercises I should be avoiding?
- Do I have any health concerns that may impact my ability to exercise?
- Is all my preventative care up to date? (National Institute on Aging, 2020)

Meet Yourself Where You Are At

You may have years of exercise under your belt, you may have taken an extended or short break, or you may have never been physically active. Regardless of where you may be on your exercise journey, start slowly and gradually build yourself up in intensity, frequency, and volume of training. The last thing we want is you to either burn out due to overactivity or injure yourself.

Start with 10 minutes a day, three times a week, or 10 minutes a day, twice a day. These chair exercises are the perfect movements to introduce, or reintroduce, you to exercise. Once you get more comfortable and fitter, you can adjust your training plan and build more activity into your lifestyle.

Warm Up and Cool Down

We must prepare our bodies for exercise. After hours of sitting or inactivity, we need to ease our muscles and joints into the physical exertion we ask them to do.

A warm-up not only prepares your body for the movements you will do in the session but also gets your blood moving around your body and ensures it will be able to handle the stress about to be placed on it.

Warm-ups can also reduce your risk of injury and let you gauge how your body feels that day so you can adjust your training program as needed. A warm-up consists of five to ten minutes of a cardio-based activity to get your heart rate elevated and blood pumping, followed by focusing on the movements or accessory movements you will be doing during your session and, if needed, a couple of gentle stretches.

Once you have completed the main exercises, performing your cooldown routine is just as important. This helps your body return to its normal pre-exercise state. It helps lower your heart rate, relax muscles, promote recovery, and prevent injury.

Dress Appropriately

You will want to be able to move throughout the exercises comfortably when working out, so choose clothing that encourages a full range of motion and keeps you cool.

Your clothing shouldn't be too tight or loose, and you should ensure that your shoes fit well and have a good grip to keep you stable. Look for clothes that are made from fabric that is breathable, moisture-wicking, and stretchable.

Drink Enough Fluids

Always drink enough water before, during, and after your workout sessions. A lack of appropriate fluid intake can lead to muscle cramps, fatigue, and headaches. Sufficient hydration also ensures that you do not get dizzy or your blood pressure doesn't drop. Drink at least 8oz of water, preferably 1 hour before exercising, and then keep sipping on your water while you work out, or take set water breaks every 15–20 minutes. Pay attention to the color of your urine: If it is pale and clear, you are most likely sufficiently hydrated.

Refrain from drinking tea or coffee before exercising, as these act as diuretics and promote fluid loss (Better Health Channel, 2015).

Get a Workout Buddy

You can either exercise with someone or join a group workout class. There are a couple of benefits to having a workout partner: You have someone to motivate you, and you have someone to watch your form and provide feedback. From a safety standpoint, there would also be others around you to spot you and assist if you feel unsteady about a particular exercise.

Set Your Goals

Once you have established where you sit on the fitness spectrum and a benchmark for where you are, you can begin setting some goals for yourself.

Based on your goals and fitness levels, we can put together a training plan to set you on the path to achieving them. Begin by focusing on short-term goals to keep you motivated and on track. Keep a log of your exercise routines and any improvements you have made, and reward yourself for accomplishing them. You are taking a big step towards your health and deserve to recognize and celebrate yourself and your progress.

How to Get Started

Depending on your previous workout experience and history, there are certain areas in your physical capacity where you are more competent than others.

After a few weeks, you notice that you are better at cardiovascular-based exercise than strength; in other words, you find it easier to jog for 15 minutes than you do to strength train. You may also be more flexible than most, but you may need help to hold your balance.

Keep track of this and adjust your plan to address these imbalances. I aim to make you a well-rounded and competent person who ticks off all the requirements of being physically fit. So when you start, you may have to give some forms of exercise more weight and focus than others.

For example, if your balance needs more work than your cardio, you could add more balance-focused training to your warm-ups and cooldowns. Choosing a tailored warm-up or cooldown is an easy way to focus on this training without adding too much extra time or effort to your workout session.

I want to highlight again that it is never too late to build muscle or improve your fitness levels. According to Weil (2022), research conducted with older adults of the average age of 87 showed an increase in thigh mass by 2.7%, an increase in walking speed by 12%, and an increase in leg strength by 113%. These are wonderful results and prove that the benefits can be profound no matter when you start.

In a similar study, participants increased their walking endurance by 38% (Weil, 2022). These studies show that not only can you continue to get stronger, but you can also improve your cardiovascular health.

As previously mentioned, you want to start slowly, which means adding more light activity to your day. Stand up every hour and walk around for five minutes. The idea is to reduce the time you are sitting or inactive. Research has shown that adding as little as 30 minutes a day can significantly impact your longevity.

It would be best if you also planned to add social and movement-based activities to your schedule in conjunction with your structured fitness plan. Go bowling or dancing, do some gardening, or organize hikes. Not only does that make you more active, but it also makes you more social, which is beneficial for your mental health.

Returning to Exercise After Injury

Unfortunately, there is always a risk of injury, whether from exercise or general day-to-day living. We are more prone to injuries or falling as we age; if we recognize this, we can counteract it and put processes in place to prevent its next occurrence. This is where exercise comes in.

According to research, exercise can help you recover from injury (Better Health Channel, 2015): So even if you suffer a physical setback, you should find ways to continue your exercise routine. The same applies to if you are recovering from surgery. Of course, before continuing exercise, you should first be cleared to work out by your doctor.

It is also important to be aware that you will not only be limited physically but may also be affected mentally. Getting injured can take its toll mentally, emotionally, and physically. It can be time-consuming and a long process, but exercise will help you recover and get through it.

The harsh truth is that, as we age, it is much harder to recover from falls, surgery, or other injuries. Our bodies have changed over the years. And I know this doesn't sound very encouraging, but you are on the right track by focusing on your health and wellness.

Understand Your Injury

Have a clear idea of your injury: You should know what kind of injury it is and why it occurred. This will set your expectations regarding recovery time, what exercise you can do, and what exercise you will need to avoid.

During this time, it is also important to know that your main focus is not to get fitter, stronger, or lose weight. Your focus is to regain functionality, reduce pain and improve your current quality of life.

Give Your Body Time to Heal but Remain Active

Depending on your injury, your healing period will vary from about six weeks to three to six months—it depends on what area was injured and whether it was tissue, ligaments, muscles, or bone. Alternatively, you may have had surgery and have a specific healing time.

Although you should rest initially, you should also remain lightly active. A simple 5-minute stretch, walk, or moving other uninjured body limbs is a great way to start. The idea is to keep your blood moving, muscles active, and your mental state in a good space.

Keep progression slow and steady—it is better to do too little exercise than too much. The last thing you want is to reinjure yourself and set yourself back in the healing process. Take one step forward each day instead of attempting three and then regress backwards.

Focus On Your Mental Health

A physical injury can cause mental setbacks as well. Aging is a time wrought with mixed feelings of both joy and apprehension. Getting injured or having to have surgery due to the changes in our aging bodies can bring forth many negative emotions.

You may feel discouraged, stressed, or disappointed—whatever you may feel, you should know that this is normal, and you can do some things to help you manage these feelings. Look to meditation or breathing techniques to help quiet your mind and reduce stress. You should also surround yourself with people who love you and care for your well-being. Keep being social and look to your community. Remember to ask for help if you need it.

Now let's look at how we can assess our fitness needs and set our goals before we begin.

Assessing Your Needs and Fitness Goals

Your goals are important: They give you something to work towards, provide a sense of accomplishment, and encourage you to get out of your comfort zone and attempt the unfamiliar with the aim of self-improvement. But if you are new to goal setting, especially with fitness goals, you may need guidance on where to start and how to reach them.

There are several ways to set goals and many ways to accomplish them. According to Better Health Channel (2012), here are some initial questions to ask yourself:

- What is your ultimate goal?
- What things can you do that will take you in the direction of your goals?
- Can you break your goals down into small manageable goals? What are they?
- Can you monitor your progress?
- Are you able to confidently adapt these goals should you need to?

You will need to be specific when setting your goals. Too broad a goal, and you will find yourself focusing on too many things instead of pinpointing your exact outcome. Be sure also to make it measurable and realistic.

The key is to set small manageable goals to increase your chances of success which keeps you motivated and progressing. Every day you can assign yourself a task that helps your fitness journey. It can be as simple as adding more water to your day. The idea is to pick things that are easy to accomplish and that you can build upon at a steady pace. Setting a reasonable timeframe should also be a consideration; it is ok for your time frame to be months from now so long as you have clear goals and plenty of checkpoints in between.

Most importantly, though, your goals need to be important and meaningful to you. What is your "why?" Your goals need to reflect what you want to accomplish and resonate with you and your wants and needs.

How are you going to achieve these goals? You have already chosen to start a chair exercise routine, but what other aspects of your life do you want to change to help you achieve your goal? Do you need to look at your nutrition and stress levels? You may also need to focus on your sleeping patterns. In what other ways can you move yourself toward your goals?

Remember to be flexible in your approach—life happens, and circumstances often change. You must be able to adapt and modify your goals as you need to and, of course, treat yourself with grace.

As with anything new, it will be challenging to adhere to these changes initially but keep being persistent. Always aim for something over nothing and progress over perfection. Celebrate your achievements no matter how small, and always make time to reflect on where you started and where you are now.

Finally, look to your community, friends, and family. They will be your biggest cheerleaders and offer support as you continue your journey.

If you are still battling to set goals or assess where you are and where you want to go, invest the time and hire a professional. A certified personal trainer can help steer you in the right direction and get you started should you feel overwhelmed. They can set up your initial assessments, set your goals, track your progress, adjust as needed, and work in conjunction with your healthcare provider to further tailor your plan.

An easy way to set up your goals based on the above recommendation is to use the acronym SMART (Sweat, 2019).

SMART goals are goals that are:

- Specific
- Measurable
- Achievable
- Relevant
- Time-bound

I have given you numerous and varied reasons why you should be excited to start your fitness journey using chair exercises to reach your health goals.

Now the time has come to start.

Get Your Chair

> Age is no barrier. It's a limitation you put on your mind.
>
> Jackie Joyner-Kersee

One of the positive benefits of this chair exercise routine is that it is so simple to integrate into your life. You do not need expensive fancy equipment, tons of space, or even to leave your house. It is very affordable, and you can work with what you have and keep things very simple.

Chair

The first thing you will need is a sturdy chair without wheels and a sturdy desk or table. These should be solid and stable with feet that will not slide on the floor.

When sitting in the chair, you should be in a position where your feet are flat on the floor, and your knees are bent at a 90° angle. The chair can have armrests if you need added support, but it can also restrict movement.

Don't worry if your chair does not meet all the specific requirements, as the beauty of chair exercises is that they can be adapted. You can use various props, such as blocks, cushions, and blankets, to adapt the chair to work for you.

Some chairs are more popular than others, but you must bear in mind the exercises you will be doing when selecting the best chair for you.

Standard Chair

A standard chair, such as a kitchen or a simple fold-up chair, can be perfect for your basic routine. One of the best chairs is a sturdy wood or metal frame that supports you and your movements without wobbling. Ensure it is the right height for your body, or use props to help you.

If you struggle with comfort, you can even use your favorite recliner. The importance is that you need to feel safe and secure in your chair.

Balance Ball Chair

These chairs offer you more of a challenge when doing a movement. They need more core strength and stability from you to balance, which will incorporate an added core workout.

Office Chair

You can use an office chair, which usually has armrests and wheels. The wheels can be a safety hazard, and I do not recommend these chairs unless you can lock the wheels in place and keep it stable.

Benches

You can even perform the exercises on your local park bench to get out of the house on a nice beautiful day. So long as whatever you are sitting on supports you and allows you the freedom of movement, you can bring your exercise routine to it.

Desk or coffee table

I recommend having a flat surface nearby for your water bottle and optional accessory exercise equipment. It could be a desk, coffee, end, or kitchen table. You will want it near enough to access your items on it but far enough away so it does not impact your workout.

Clothing and Shoes

We touched briefly on clothing in a previous section and discussed how it impacts our safety. Depending on the movements and temperature, we will also need to have the appropriate attire to work out in.

Shoe selection is also a significant decision; according to Living Maples (2021), exercise can cause foot issues such as plantar fasciitis unless we use the correct footwear to support our feet. In addition, shoes that are not supportive can pinch our feet and cause blisters and calluses, which would make for a very unpleasant exercise experience.

Select shoes that are lightweight and made of breathable fabric. You want shoes that won't put added pressure on certain parts of your feet, as these could irritate bunions. Although you want them to be soft and easy on your feet, you do not want to sacrifice support and stability. Shoes should support the ankle and arches of your feet.

Optional Equipment

There are certain other accessories that you can use to customize and change your workout routine. Usually, these will make the program and movements more challenging as you are ready to progress. Two of the main ones are dumbbells and resistance bands. I have added a section at the end of the book titled-Optional Amazon Purchases with links to where you can find the equipment to be purchased.

Dumbbells

A pair of dumbbells can be used to progress once you have become proficient at the arm exercises and are looking to make your workouts more challenging. Adding weight is called progressive overload, the process of adding difficulty to a movement to make you stronger. You can do this by changing tempos or increasing the number of repetitions in your exercise routines.

If you decide to use weights, you must pick the appropriate weight. You want to use a challenging weight that allows you to keep good form and perform your allocated repetitions with slight ease or struggle.

At first, you can purchase a pair of light dumbbells before looking to get any heavier weights—the light dumbbells will let you progress quite sufficiently for a couple of months.

Resistance Bands

Resistance bands come in different varieties, such as loop, tube, or flat bands; we are interested in Flat bands. Flat bands are flat elastic bands made of either natural latex or Thermoplastic Elastomer (TPE) used for physical therapy with various lengths, colors, and resistance values. They are fantastic workout tools because they are portable, affordable, and easy on your joints. They offer the user a great way to do a low-impact workout that still builds strength.

Along with supporting your stabilizer muscles, resistance bands also help create strength in our larger muscles and joints. They are great at helping you maintain and increase your bone density.

Please check your resistance bands for wear before each use; elastics can degrade over time, become dry, brittle, and possibly crack and break if not stored out of UV rays.

Hand Exercise Balls

Hand exercise balls are a great way to relieve stress and tension in the hands, wrists, and forearms. They are beneficial for gently working through your arthritis and carpal tunnel to ease and relax your nerves while strengthening your surrounding tissue. Hand exercise balls come in various shapes, from round balls to oval or egg-shaped, with different colors and resistance values. The egg-shaped exercise balls are best for our hand squeeze exercise as the egg shape helps apply an even pressure inside your hand when gripped. Some hand exercise balls can be cooled or warmed to provide soothing or numbing nerves while providing the same resistance values.

Workout Gloves

When using weights, your hands can take a knock, and you may develop calluses. You may also need the comfort, support, and grip that wearing gloves may provide.

Some gloves can also provide wrist support, usually by providing a band around your wrist that you can tighten to offer stability while working with the weights.

At-home Equipment Alternatives

You may not have the budget or means to spend on the above equipment, which is perfectly fine. You most likely already have plenty of items in your home that you use to make the exercises more challenging.

Water bottles or milk jugs

Water bottles and gallon water or milk jugs are not just for rehydrating yourself but can also be used as alternatives to dumbbell weights. Water bottles are fairly easy to grip and move around with but large. Gallon jugs come with a carrying handle which can be easier to grip but, depending on how full, can put additional strain on your wrist downward. With every 16 oz of water equalling 1 pound of weight, you can quickly and easily scale from 0.5 lbs for a half-full water 16oz plastic water bottle to 8 lbs full gallon jug just with the amount of water you add.

Rolled Towel

Towels come in many sizes that you can fold and roll into the right shape for your grip for squeezing. They are an excellent at-home alternative to exercise balls that can also be heated or cooled depending on your need for soothing or numbing stubborn arthritis when exercising.

Safety Tips

While I have given you options for various equipment that you can use to add challenges to your workout, known as progressive overload, I want to talk about safety and form. Form refers to how well we perform throughout the movement of the exercise. Our goal is always to move through the motions with control and confidence before taxing our bodies with additional challenges. Try each exercise once, without additional equipment, moving slowly with control through the motions, and assess how it feels.

- Did you feel shaky or struggle at any point?
- Did you feel like you were on the verge of losing your balance at any point?
- Did you feel any new or unusual pain or discomfort?

If you feel any of these issues, it is essential to pause and address them before proceeding. Remember, the goal isn't to rush through the exercises but to perform them safely and effectively. It's perfectly okay to modify the exercise and only take the movement as far as you feel safe with your current physical state. If any exercise causes consistent discomfort or pain, it may be best to avoid it until you can consult with your healthcare provider.

We only want to add difficulty to our basic movements once we have successfully mastered our form. I also want you to take your time and not feel rushed to add more challenges to your workout. Slow and steady is how we will progress. We should aim to take small jumps every few weeks or months. We do not want to risk injury or burnout.

It is also important to remember from a physical and mental standpoint that you may be unable to jump to the next stage at each suggested increase—progressive overload is not linear. Just because you are not improving at the rate you envisioned for yourself does not mean that you are not getting stronger and improving. Sometimes you might have an off week and need a little more rest. Keep the vision of continuously improving, but only move up your progress in progressive overload when you move through the exercise with good form, confidence, and ease.

How to Progress and Adapt Your Workouts

As you become fitter and stronger, you will inevitably need to make your program more challenging. There are various ways to do this. Some of the exercises we included in this book have modifications listed, including versions with weights, tempos, and bands.

The following section will go into detail as to how you can progress your program. I have allocated eight repetitions and one set for each movement or a minimum of 15 seconds for some movements. While this starting point might be good for most, you can pick whatever starting point works for you and build from there. You might be surprised at how much you can get out of chair exercises, as there is so much room to grow from just sets and reps in the beginning. Further increase in your results can be gained in your exercises using more advanced techniques such as tempo, pauses, or weights.

As we get deeper into our workout program, we will look to manipulate the following variables to illicit progressive overload throughout the weeks. These variables that we can work with are:

- frequency
- intensity
- volume
- rest period
- tempo (Provectus Physiotherapy & Health Services, 2022)

Progressive overload refers to the stress you put on your body when exercising. To see results, we need to add slightly more stress to our bodies by making our workout program more challenging over time.

Each session, your body will adapt to the stimulus, then you add more, and it adapts to that, thus becoming stronger.

When managed and executed well, you can guarantee that you will continue to see favorable results as time progresses. We do not need to add sets and reps or weights to your program weekly, but it can, and should, take place over weeks to ensure you are safe and injury free.

Frequency

Frequency refers to the amount of workouts that you do in a certain period. For instance, if you are just starting and are new to exercising, you may want to begin with two sessions a week.

Continue for two to three weeks until your body adjusts, and then add another session. Continue with this until you reach your frequency goals.

Here is an example plan based on frequency:

- Week one: Finish two workouts.
- Week two: Finish two workouts.
- Week three: Finish three workouts.
- Week four: Finish three workouts.
- Week four: Finish four workouts.
- Week five: Finish four workouts.
- Week six: Finish five workouts.

Intensity

Intensity refers to the process of adding weight to your movements. You could aim to go up in weight every four weeks or stick to a progression where you find it very easy to lift a weight between 8 to 12 repetitions. So when you are ready to lift heavier, look for a weight that gives you a challenge for 8 repetitions.

And, of course, it's very important that you only increase weight if your form allows you to. Moving well is far more beneficial than moving load.

Here is an example of a plan that utilizes intensity for progressive overload:

- Week one: Perform 12 bicep curls with 2 lbs.
- Week two: Perform 12 bicep curls with 2 lbs.
- Week three: Perform 12 bicep curls with 2 lbs.
- Week four: Perform 8 bicep curls with 3 lbs.
- Week five: Perform 8 bicep curls with 3 lbs.
- Week six: Perform 8 bicep curls with 3 lbs.

On week 4, I added weight as the 12 reps felt relatively easy and needed a challenge.

Volume

Volume refers to the number of repetitions. If you do three sets of eight repetitions, your total volume is 24 repetitions.

Here is an example of a plan that utilizes volume for progressive overload:

- Week one: Perform 10 calf raises.
- Week two: Perform 10 calf raises.
- Week three: Perform 12 calf raises.
- Week four: Perform 12 calf raises.
- Week five: Perform 12 calf raises.
- Week six: Perform 14 calf raises.

Rest Period

The rest period refers to the amount of time that you rest between sets or movements.

For instance, you could do three sets of calf raises with a rest of 90 seconds between each set. You could reduce your rest time to a minute in the following workout session.

The rest time you need is determined based on how much time your body needs to recover from an exercise while still maintaining good form.

Here is an example of a plan that utilizes rest for progressive overload:

- Week one: Perform 12 calf raises, rest 90 seconds.
- Week two: Perform 12 calf raises, rest 90 seconds.
- Week three: Perform 12 calf raises, rest 1 minute.
- Week four: Perform 12 calf raises, rest 1 minute.
- Week five: Perform 12 calf raises, rest 1 minute.
- Week six: Perform 12 calf raises, rest 1 minute.

Tempo

Tempo refers to the speed at which you complete each movement, also known as the muscles' time under tension.

Studies have found that when you slow down your movements, you require more stabilization, balance, power, agility, and strength to complete the task. Slowing down the movement helps target the smaller muscles that stabilize and control your finer movements. By changing the tempo, you can increase the strength of these smaller muscle groups so they do not fatigue as fast throughout the day.

Usually, we will slow down the motion of the movement or pause for a moment at the end of the range of motion to elicit this stimulus.

It is written as follows: 8 Bicep Curls at a 3242 tempo.

Each number is how many seconds you should take from one movement to the next, as so.

- 3 seconds to curl your arm up from the resting position to your shoulder.
- 2-second hold with your arm muscles tight at the top of the position.
- 4 seconds slowly releasing your curl to the bottom resting position.
- 2-second rest before starting the next Bicep Curl.

Here is an example of a plan that utilizes tempo for progressive overload.

- Week one: Perform 8 Bicep curls at a 2231 tempo
- Week two: Perform 8 Bicep curls at a 2231 tempo
- Week three: Perform 8 Bicep curls at a 2231 tempo
- Week four: Perform 8 Bicep curls at a 3242 tempo
- Week five: Perform 8 Bicep curls at a 3242 tempo
- Week six: Perform 8 Bicep curls at a 3242 tempo

Combining Techniques

You can also combine progressive overload techniques as you progress. For instance, if you have been adding repetitions to your program and now want to progress even further, you can add tempo to those reps.

You may need to lower the number of reps, but the tempo will ensure you are still adding stimulus to your program and providing progressive overload.

Here is an example of a plan that utilizes reps and tempo for progressive overload.

- Week one: Perform 10 calf raises.
- Week two: Perform 10 calf raises.
- Week three: Perform 10 calf raises.
- Week four: Perform 8 calf raises at a 2321 tempo.
- Week five: Perform 8 calf raises at a 2321 tempo.
- Week six: Perform 8 calf raises at a 2321 tempo.

As you get more advanced, you can begin to use more than two protocols. You can be as creative as you like. As you can see, the further into your workout routine, the more interesting and customizable you can get; therefore, it also helps to keep a record and workout journal to keep track of your progress and changes.

Here is an example of a plan that utilizes weight, tempo, and rest periods for progressive overload:

- Week one: Perform 10 bicep curls with 2 lbs at a 3231 tempo with a rest for 90 seconds.
- Week two: Perform 10 bicep curls with 2 lbs at a 3231 tempo with a rest for 90 seconds.

- Week three: Perform 8 bicep curls with 2 lbs at a 3232 tempo with a rest for 1 minute.
- Week four: Perform 8 bicep curls with 2 lbs at a 3232 tempo with a rest for 1 minute.
- Week five: Perform 8 bicep curls with 3 lbs at a 3231 tempo with a rest for 90 seconds.
- Week six: Perform 8 bicep curls with 3 lbs at a 3231 tempo with a rest for 90 seconds.

Now that we have chosen our chair and understand how to modify the exercises over time, let's get warmed up.

Warming up

> We do not stop exercising because we grow old- we grow old because we stop exercising.
>
> Dr. Kenneth Cooper

You may feel that you do not need to warm up since you will essentially be exercising sitting down for most of these exercises, but do not be fooled by thinking that these are too simple to require a sufficient warm-up.

There are several reasons why warming up is important.

Raises Body Temperature and Prepares Your Muscles

Your warm-up will prepare your body for activity by warming up your muscles and increasing your heart rate. This also allows your muscles to expand and contract efficiently, thus increasing their elasticity. It also gets your oxygen-rich blood pumping throughout your body to your extremities.

Your warm-up also prepares your joints and tendons to be able to extend comfortably through their full range of motion, and the increased flexibility will help you complete the movements more efficiently and safely. This has long-term benefits besides warming you up for your current workout—the long-term flexibility will last long after your workout.

Prepares You Mentally to Exercise

A good warm-up gets you into the headspace to exercise. It can be tough to get motivated on some days, but starting a warm-up and moving through the motions makes you eager to continue and complete your workout.

On days when I do not feel like exercising, I tell myself just to put on my shoes and do a quick warm-up and take it from there. In these instances, I usually end up doing the whole exercise session finding myself grateful that I pushed myself to start the warm-up.

Use this time to focus and think about your goals. It is a great time to assess how far you have come, how far you are going, and how proactive you currently are about your health and wellness.

Improves Performance

The point of exercise is to make you fitter and stronger and to ensure you are moving efficiently. It is pointless for us to go through the motions to get the work done. While it can be easy just to set up, work out, and move on with our day (particularly if it has been long and tiring), we must treat our workout routines seriously.

When you warm up, you practice the movements beforehand and can tweak your form or change the movement if needed. It also gives you a chance to work on any coordination issues. Warm-ups also allow you time to go through your program for the day and adapt it if needed. For example, your knee may be a bit tender, so you choose to do an upper-body workout instead.

To get the best results, we need to perform at our best. A good warm-up provides this both physically and mentally.

Accessory or Balance Work

Your warm-up is part of your exercise routine, which can be used to work on different movements and exercises that are not part of your primary exercise routine but are beneficial to have in your program. Movements such as balance work, stretching, or other accessory exercises can be incorporated to save time during your sessions and work as a warm-up session, effectively creating a well-rounded, time-saving routine.

Prevents Injury

Injury prevention is the primary goal of any warm-up. We want to prepare the body and mind and prevent any risk of injury. The goal is to decrease any unnecessary stress or tension on the tendons, ligaments, joints, or bones.

It also benefits your post-workout recovery and can prevent delayed onset muscle soreness, or DOMS.

Please remember as we go through the following warm-up routines that you should never push the movement into any discomfort or pain.

General Warm-ups

Warm-up Routine One

1. Begin by sitting upright in your chair with your shoulders down and back.
   2. Place your hands on your thighs.

2. Inhale and, as you slowly exhale, look over your left shoulder,

keeping your torso facing forward and only moving from your neck.

3. Return your head to the center.
4. Inhale and, as you slowly exhale, look over your right shoulder, keeping your torso facing forward and only moving from your neck.
5. Return your head to the center.
6. Inhale and slowly tilt your head upwards, looking at the ceiling.
7. Exhale and slowly lower your head, bringing your chin to your chest.
8. Repeat this sequence.
9. Inhale, shrug your shoulders towards your ears, and roll them backward, creating small circles.
10. Repeat for five rotations.
11. Raise your arms in front of your body, keeping them straight and holding a fist with your hands. They should be in line with your chest.
12. Inhale and pull them back towards your chest, then exhale and push them out straight in front of you.
13. Repeat three times.
14. Lower your hands to the side of you, your palms facing your

thighs, and your thumbs pointed forward.

15. Inhale and raise your arms straight in front of you at a 90° angle. Exhale and lower them back to your sides, keeping your arms straight and elbows locked out.
16. Inhale and raise your arms to extend overhead as far as possible while keeping them straight. At the top, stretch towards the ceiling and wiggle your fingers for a few seconds.
17. Exhale and lower them back to your sides, keeping your arms straight and elbows locked out.
18. Return your arms to the side, your palms facing forward, and your thumbs pointed outwards.
19. Inhale and raise your arms out to the side of you to a 90° angle. Exhale and gently lower them to the starting position.
20. Inhale and raise your arms out to the side of you and extend all the way overhead.
21. At the top, stretch towards the ceiling and wiggle your fingers for a few seconds. Exhale and gently lower them to the starting position.
22. Repeat for three repetitions.
23. Raise your arms to 90° again. Gently circle your arms forward, ensuring your shoulders are down and back.
24. Repeat for five rotations, and then rotate your arms backward

for five rotations.

25. Lower your hands to the side of you, your palms facing your thighs, and your thumbs pointed forward.
26. Inhale and raise your arms overhead as far as possible while keeping them straight.
27. Keeping your arms straight, gently lower them, but this time lower them from your back and hips, leaning all the way forward as you bring them to your shins or toes. Exhale as you do so.
28. Slowly raise them back overhead.
29. Repeat for five repetitions, and hold this position for five seconds on the last repetition at the bottom of the movement.
30. Place your arms straight at your side with your palms facing forward.
31. Curl your arms upwards and touch your shoulders with your fingertips.
32. Lower them back down and repeat for three more repetitions.
33. Raise your arms in front of you at chest height.
34. Rotate your wrists outwards for five repetitions.
35. Rotate your wrists inwards for five repetitions.
36. Scoot yourself so that you are now sitting up against the back of your chair. Keep your shoulders engaged back and down.

37. Inhale and lift and straighten your left leg by bending at the knee. Hold this position for a few seconds.

38. Exhale, slowly lower your leg to the floor and repeat on the other side. Repeat for six repetitions on each side.

39. Move to the middle of the chair, keeping your legs at a 90° angle, and lift your leg past your knee.

40. Repeat on the other side and alternate for six sets.

41. Move yourself to the front of the chair, place your hands on your knees, and ensure you are still sitting up tall with your shoulders back and down.

42. Inhale and raise your feet onto your toes, exhale, and lower them back down. Repeat for three repetitions.

43. Remaining at the front of your chair, shift your legs slightly forward.

44. Raise your toes so that your feet are now on your heels. Repeat for three repetitions.

45. Return your legs so your feet are back in line with your knees. Step out your left leg to the left side, and return to the middle.

46. Step out your right leg to the right side. Alternate on each leg for three repetitions on each side.

47. Lift and straighten your left leg by bending at the knee. Hold your leg straight up and flex your foot. Point your toes forward

and then point them backward.

48. Repeat for three reps and swap legs.

49. Lift your left leg and raise your foot. Rotate from your ankle in a circular direction clockwise for five repetitions. Rotate from your ankle in a circular direction anticlockwise for five repetitions. Return your foot to the ground.

50. Lift your right leg and raise your foot. Rotate from your ankle in a circular direction clockwise for five repetitions. Rotate from your ankle in a circular direction anticlockwise for five repetitions. Return your foot to the ground.

51. Sit back in your chair and raise your arms into a boxing position in front of your chest. Punch your arms forward in a boxing motion for 30 seconds.

52. Move forward in your chair, placing your feet under your knees. Raise your left leg so your knee goes just above your thigh in a marching motion.

53. Repeat with the other leg and swing your arms at the same time. Alternate your marching steps for 15 seconds.

Warm-up Routine Two

1. Begin by sitting upright in your chair with your shoulders down and back.

2. Place your hands on your thighs.

3. Inhale and, as you exhale, slowly look over your left shoulder, keeping your torso facing forward and only moving from your neck.

4. Return your head to the center.

5. Inhale and, as you exhale, slowly look over your right shoulder, keeping your torso facing forward and only moving from your neck.

6. Return your head to the center.

7. Place your hands across your chest, keeping your back straight and upright. Exhale and gently twist to the left, moving your whole torso as you do so.

8. Return to the middle and, as you exhale, gently twist to the right. Repeat for six repetitions.

9. Shift yourself so you are sitting up against the back of your chair. Keep your shoulders engaged back and down.

10. Inhale and lift and straighten your left leg by bending at the knee. Hold this position for a few seconds.

11. Exhale, slowly lower it to the floor and repeat on the other side.

Repeat for six repetitions on each side.

12. Shift yourself so you are now sitting at the front of your chair. Keep your shoulders engaged back and down.
13. Slide your left foot in front of you until fully extended, then slide your foot back under your chair. Repeat for five repetitions.
14. Swap sides and repeat.
15. Lift your left leg and raise your foot. Rotate from your ankle in a circular direction clockwise for five repetitions. Rotate from your ankle in a circular direction anticlockwise for five repetitions. Return your foot to the ground.
16. Lift your right leg and raise your foot. Rotate from your ankle in a circular direction clockwise for five repetitions. Rotate from your ankle in a circular direction anticlockwise for five repetitions. Return your foot to the ground.
17. Move forward in your chair, placing your feet under your knees. Raise your left leg so your knee goes just above your thigh in a marching motion.
18. Repeat with the other leg and swing your arms at the same time. Alternate your marching steps for 30 seconds.

Warm-up Routine Three

1. Begin by sitting upright in your chair with your shoulder blades down and back.
2. Your feet should be flat on the floor.
3. Inhale, bring your arms up and place your hands behind your head at the base of your skull.
4. Intertwine your fingers and let your head rest in the cups of your hands. Inhale and turn your head slightly towards the ceiling.
5. Inhale and gently bend to the right. Your right elbow should rise to the ceiling, and your left elbow should drop toward the ground.
6. Stay here for a two-second count and return to a neutral position.
7. Repeat on the other side.
8. Alternate between left and right for six repetitions.
9. Move towards the front of your chair, giving you space behind you.
10. Place your palms on your lower back and hips.
11. As you exhale, gently arch your back and push your hips forward while carefully bending your neck backward as you look toward the ceiling.

12. Hold this position for five breaths.
13. Return to your starting position.
14. Stay seated forward in your chair and reach your hands backward, interlacing your fingers. If this is a difficult position for you, then grab hold of your wrists or forearms.
15. Take a deep breath in and roll your shoulders up and back.
16. As you breathe out, straighten your arms behind you.
17. Hold this position for three full breaths and return to neutral.
18. Keeping your arms clasped and behind you, gently bend forward from your waist.
19. Your arms should be rising behind you as you do so.
20. Bend down as far as comfortable without collapsing into the stretch.
21. Return to your seated position with your shoulders back and down and your feet planted under you at a 90° angle.
22. Place your hands on your thighs with your fingers pointed towards each other. Your palms rotated so that the heels of your palms are pointed outwards.
23. Press into your thighs and, as you inhale, arch your back and bend your neck backward, bringing your gaze towards the ceiling. Think about gently pushing your buttocks backward.

24. Inhale, roll your shoulders forward and draw your belly button towards your spine. Gently drop your chin towards your chest while maintaining the pressure of your palms on your thighs.

25. Repeat this alternating sequence three to five times.

26. Return to your starting position, sitting upright in your chair.

27. As you inhale, bring your arms over your head.

28. Exhale and gently turn your torso to the right. Put your left hand on the outside of your left knee and your right hand in a position that feels most comfortable to you. You will feel a gentle twist in your spine.

29. Hold this position for three to five breaths as you sink deeper into the stretch.

30. Return to your neutral position and repeat on the other side.

Targeted Warm-ups

Ankle and Leg Warm-up Routine

1. Begin by standing up tall next to your chair for support. Keep your shoulder blades back and down.
2. Hold onto the chair's backrest for support and lift your left leg so that you are standing on your right leg.
3. Move your left leg out to the side of you and gently rotate from your hips in a clockwise direction. Repeat for 20 repetitions in this direction.
4. Repeat for 20 repetitions in an anticlockwise direction.
5. Switch legs and repeat on the other side in both directions.
6. Return to your neutral position with your arms at your side.
7. Rotating from your shoulders and keeping your arms straight, swing them forward for 20 rotations.
8. Swing them backward for 20 rotations.
9. Return to a neutral position and lift your arms to align with your shoulders with your palms facing the floor.
10. Swing them inwards towards each other so that they cross in front of your chest. Swing them back out the side.
11. Repeat for 20 repetitions.

12. Stand next to your chair using the backrest for support if needed.

13. Lift your left leg as high as possible, bringing your knee up towards your chest. Exhale and, using your arm, pull your knee towards you as your other arm provides balance. Hold for a few seconds before lowering.

14. Repeat on the other side.

15. Return to a neutral standing position.

16. Take a small step forward and place your heel on the ground. Roll your foot gently forward as you step so that you roll onto your toes and the ball of your foot.

17. Rise as high as possible onto your toes.

18. Repeat on the other side.

19. Alternate this step for five repetitions on each foot.

Core Warm-up Routine

1. Begin by sitting upright in the middle of your chair with your shoulders down and back.
2. Move your feet so that they are slightly in front of you.
3. Bring both of your hands across your chest.
4. Exhale and lean backward until your back lightly touches the back of your chair.
5. Inhale and lean forward until you are sitting up straight again.
6. Repeat for five repetitions.
7. Return to sitting upright in the middle of your chair and lean backward, keeping your back straight.
8. Inhale and bring your knees up towards your chest.
9. Exhale and lower them back down in front of you.
10. Repeat for five repetitions.
11. Return to sitting upright in the middle of your chair and place your hands on the hand rests.
12. Inhale and, on your exhale, move your feet forward so your legs are extended, your heels are on the floor, and your toes are raised to the ceiling.
13. Inhale and draw your feet back towards you so your feet are

under your chair. You should be on your toes with your heels pointed toward the ceiling.

14. Repeat for five repetitions.

Now that you feel warmed up, let us move on to our ankle and leg exercises.

Ankle and Leg Exercises

> The best day to start exercising is today. Tomorrow can turn into weeks, months, or years.
>
> Mark Dilworth

Our feet and legs carry us through life: from our first precarious steps to dances at our children's weddings or to our afternoon strolls. Our feet go through a lot, and most of us do not stop to think about them when considering building strength. We tend to focus on the other more popular body parts and muscle groups and need to recognize the importance of having strong feet and ankles.

Providing our bodies with a solid foundation and base will ensure that we protect our joints, bones, and tendons as we age. We can mitigate some of the adverse effects of aging on our lower extremities and keep the rest of our body functioning optimally; after all, they are all connected, and one weak link in the chain affects the others.

Changes that occur can cause stability problems, which can cause hip, knee, and back issues. The most common problems associated with aging and our feet are those related to skin, connective tissues, joints, nails, and blood circulation (Moyer, 2020).

Arthritis

According to Moyer (2020), arthritis or osteoarthritis affects about 10% of men and 13% of women over 60. Osteoarthritis affects the joints in the foot, particularly the ankle joint, big toe, and subtalar joint, which is located by your heel. Arthritis can cause pain and stiffness, which can impair movement.

Edema

Edema is the medical term for circulatory problems that cause tissue swelling. This swelling is caused by fluid retention, and the main culprit is usually the hormonal changes that occur during aging. Edema can occur on one leg or both.

Flat Feet

As your ligaments stretch and lengthen, you may develop flat feet. You may find that your arch will begin to flatten, and you will experience more pain along your midfoot, resulting in some inflammation.

Flat feet also impact the hip, knee, and lower back, with some adverse effects being pain and discomfort in this area.

All these issues can lead to balance and stability woes as they progress.

Tendons Tighten

Our tendons, which connect our bones to our muscles, begin to tighten as we age because the water content in our tendons decreases.

This limits the range of motion in our feet, toes, and ankles, which limits our ability to flex them properly.

The result is that our feet flatten out, and our gait changes to compensate. The Achilles tendon is the most common area where this occurs (Moyer, 2020).

Ankle and Leg Exercises

Ankle Circles

This exercise engages the smaller muscles in the feet that do not get much attention during the day or other exercises. In addition, ankle circles increase circulation to your lower extremities and improve the mobility and flexibility of your feet. By focusing on the controlled movement of the ankle, this exercise can also improve your balance and proprioception, which is your body's ability to sense its position and movement in space. This is particularly important for preventing falls and maintaining balance as we age.

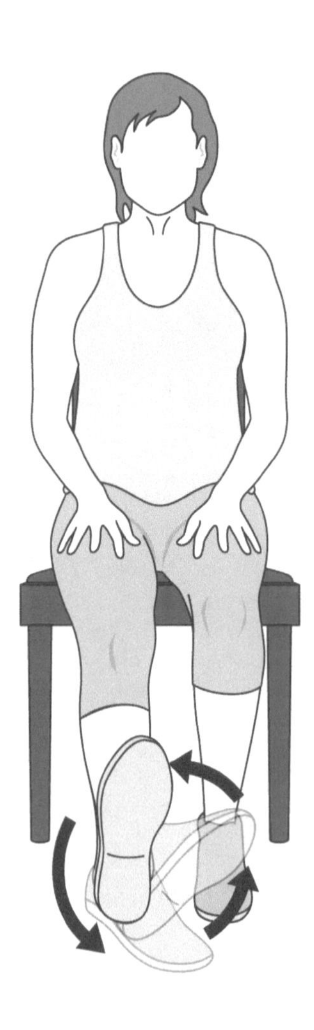

1. Begin by sitting upright in your chair with your shoulders down and back.
2. Lift your left foot off the ground.
3. Pretend that your big toe is a pen, and you are drawing a circle with it in a clockwise direction.
4. Rotate clockwise for 10 rotations.
5. Repeat in a counterclockwise direction for 10 rotations.
6. Lower your left foot back down to the ground.
7. Repeat 10 clockwise and counterclockwise rotations for the right foot.

Target: We want to explore our ankle joint's full range of motion during this exercise.

Making it easier: Lower the reps and feel free to take small breaks and rest your leg if holding it up for all the repetitions proves too challenging. Once rested, continue and finish the reps.

Adding difficulty: Increase the volume of reps or write your name and surname instead of performing circles.

Hip Marching

This exercise engages core stability and coordination while improving hip joint mobility and strengthens your hip flexors essential to walking and climbing stairs.

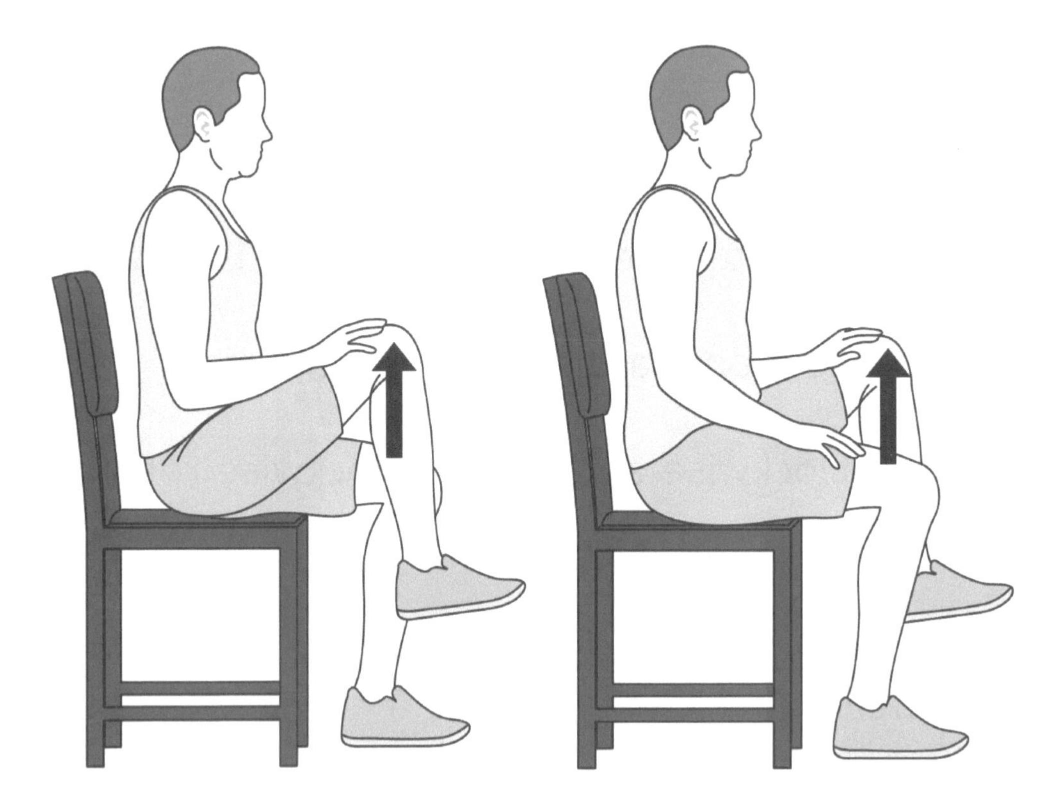

1. Begin by sitting upright in your chair with your shoulders down and back.

2. Place your feet directly under your knees.

3. Raise your right knee, keeping it bent so your foot lifts off the ground. Raise it as high as you feel comfortable.

4. Return your foot to the ground.

5. Repeat with the other leg.

6. Alternate this marching movement for 1 minute.

Target: Smooth and controlled movement as you alternate raising your knees while concentrating on keeping your back straight as you maintain your balance and coordination.

Making it easier: Limit how high you lift your knee or use your hands to help guide and raise your knees.

Adding difficulty: Add resistance by pushing down on your raising knee with your hand as you lift, holding a weight over your knee, or looping a resistance band around your leg just above your knees. You can also slow down the exercise to focus on increasing your stability and control or speed up the tempo to increase your heart rate and cardiovascular fitness.

Seated Leg and Hip Extensions

This exercise strengthens the quadriceps muscles in the front of your thighs.

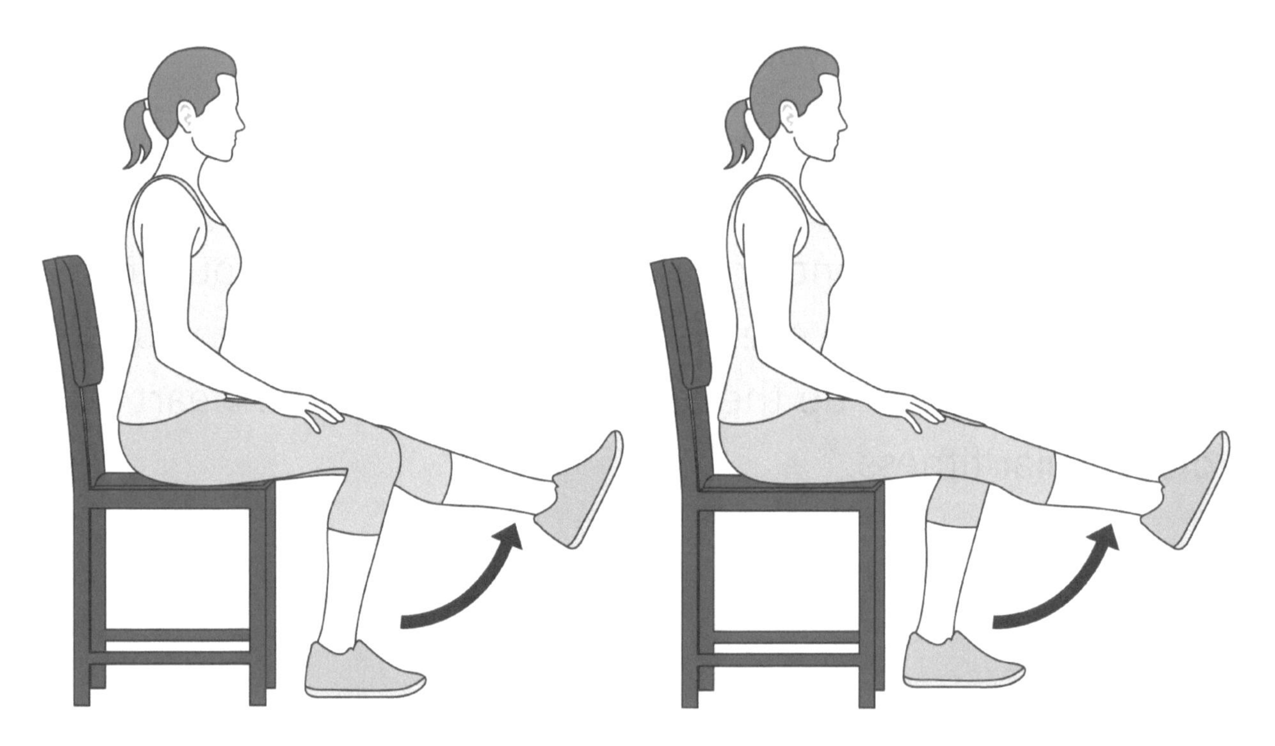

1. Begin by sitting upright in your chair with your shoulders down and back.

2. Place your feet directly under your knees.

3. Raise your left foot so your leg is straight out directly in front of you.

4. Lower your left foot back down to the resting position.

5. Raise your right foot so your leg is straight out directly in front of you.

6. Lower your left foot back down to the resting position.

7. Continue to alternate each leg for 8 reps each.

Target: We want to move smoothly, gently raising our lower legs and feet up to straight and down again with control.

Making it easier: Decrease your range of motion by only raising your leg and foot as far as you feel comfortable.

Adding difficulty: Try adding a tempo, such as 3432, or increasing the volume of reps.

Seated Hip and Knee Extension

This exercise combines hip marching and leg and hip extension movements to build strength and coordination for bicycle exercise in the dynamic core exercise section.

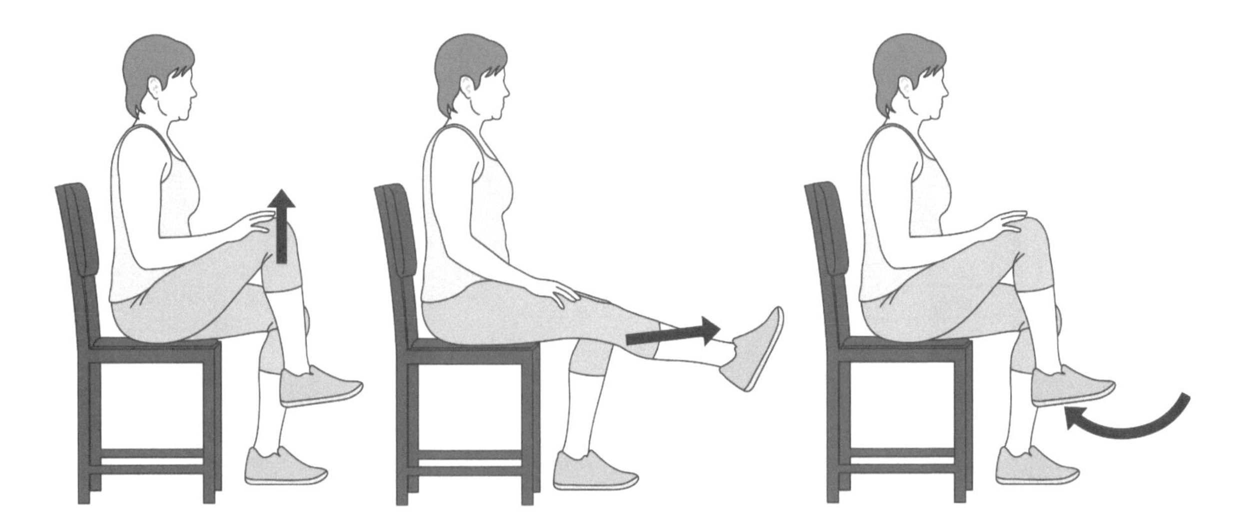

1. Begin by sitting upright in your chair with your shoulders down and back.
2. Place your feet directly under your knees.
3. Raise your right knee, keeping it bent so your foot lifts off the ground.
4. Extend your foot forward as you lower your knee to straighten your leg.
5. Pull back your foot towards you as you raise your knee.
6. Lower your knee and return your foot to the ground.
7. Repeat for your left leg.

8. Perform alternately raising, extending, and returning your leg to the resting position for 6 reps each leg.

Target: Smooth and controlled motion as you transition through the movements. Focus on where your foot is moving through the space.

Making it easier: Reduce the extent of the movement to where you feel comfortable.

Adding difficulty: Add a tempo, such as 223322, where 2 seconds would be raising your knee, 2 seconds extending your leg, 3 seconds holding, 3 seconds pulling your leg back, 2 seconds returning your foot to the floor, and 2 seconds rest. You can also increase your volume of reps.

Standing Knee Flexion

This exercise strengthens your hamstrings at the back of your thigh and helps your balance and coordination on one foot, which is essential to walking and climbing.

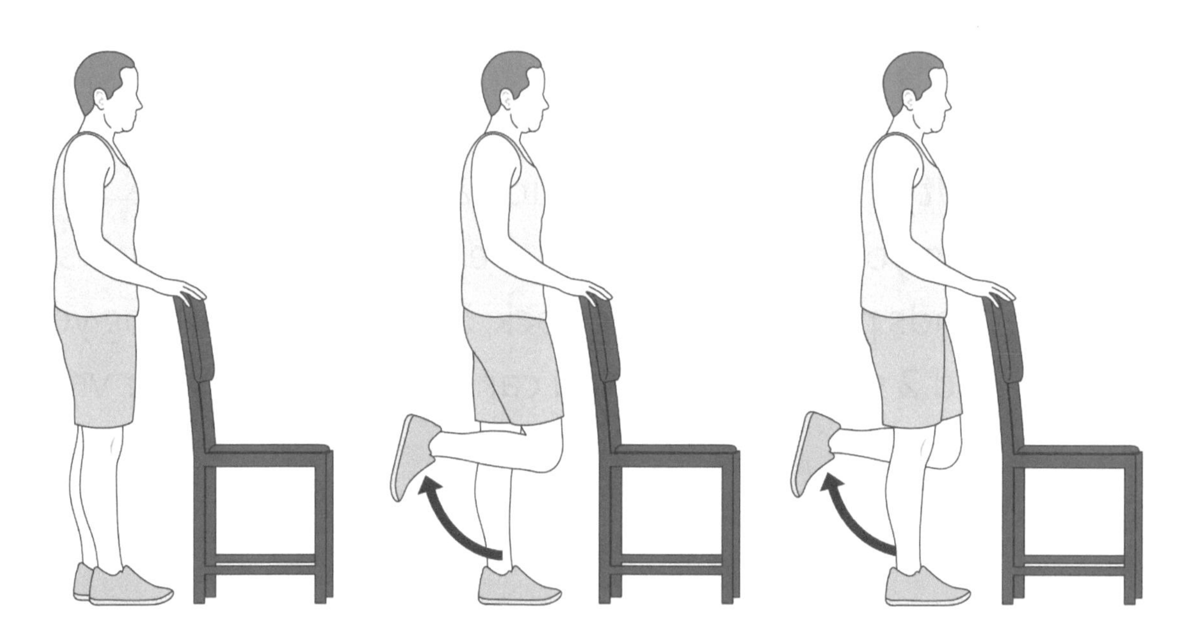

Safety Moment: Please be wary of maintaining your balance during this exercise. Go only as far as you feel comfortable—we are not looking to push ourselves into uncomfortable or unsafe positions.

1. Stand tall behind your chair, keeping your feet close together.
2. Place your hands on the chair's backrest for support. Leaning on the chair as much as necessary.
3. Bend your right knee lifting your foot behind you, bringing your heel up as high as you feel comfortable.
4. Return your right foot to the ground to the resting position.
5. Bend your left knee lifting your foot behind you, bringing your heel up as high as you feel comfortable.

6. Return your left foot to the ground to the resting position.

7. Repeat for 8 leg lifts each.

Target: Always verify that your chair is stable and will not move on you during this exercise. Focus on keeping your core strong and your balance in control throughout the exercise, only moving within your comfort zone.

Making it easier: Limit your range of motion by only sliding your foot back and rolling up onto the ball of your foot until you feel comfortable lifting your foot off the ground.

Adding difficulty: Increase your range of motion, aiming to raise your heel as close to your buttocks as possible. Add resistance in the form of a resistance band, stepping on the free ends of the band and pulling the flat of the band wrap around your heel as you lift it up.

Ankle Pumps

This exercise enhances the ankle joint mobility and range of motion. It improves blood circulation to prevent clots and deep vein thrombosis (DVT) and reduces swellings from edema.

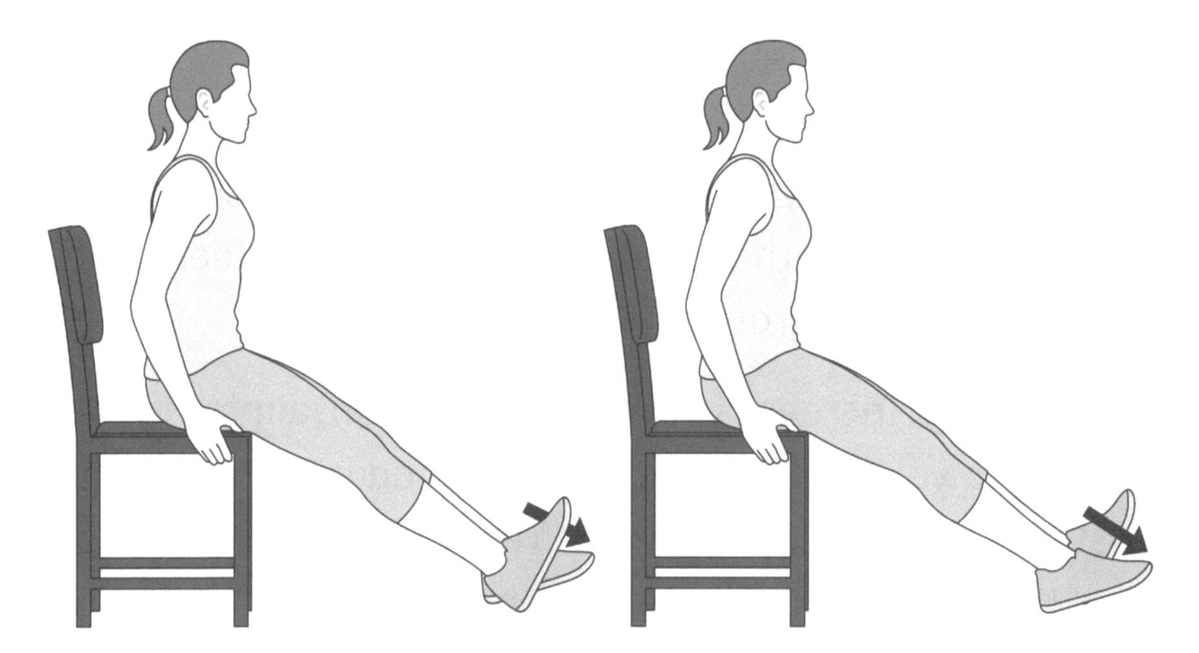

1. Begin by sitting close to the front of the chair.
2. Hold the sides of the chair seat for support.
3. Extend your legs out straight with your heels resting on the ground.
4. Flex your ankles so your left toes point down and your right toes point up.
5. Flex your ankles so your right toes point down and your left toes point up.
6. Alternate flexing your ankles for 8 reps up and down.

Target: We want smooth and controlled movement as we flex between each motion and expand our ankles' mobility range.

Making it easier: To simplify the movement, move both ankles together instead of oppositionally or perform the movement with just one leg at a time.

Adding difficulty: Lift your heels instead of allowing them to rest on the ground while performing the exercise. You can also add resistance by holding on to the ends of the resistance band while kneading the resistance band with the tips of your toes. You can also add a steady even tempo of 2222 with 2 seconds between cycling from one movement to the other and then holding for 2 seconds before moving again.

Seated Calf Raises

This exercise increases our ability to improve balance and coordination while strengthing our calf muscles which are vital to our stability and stretching up to reach things in the cupboards.

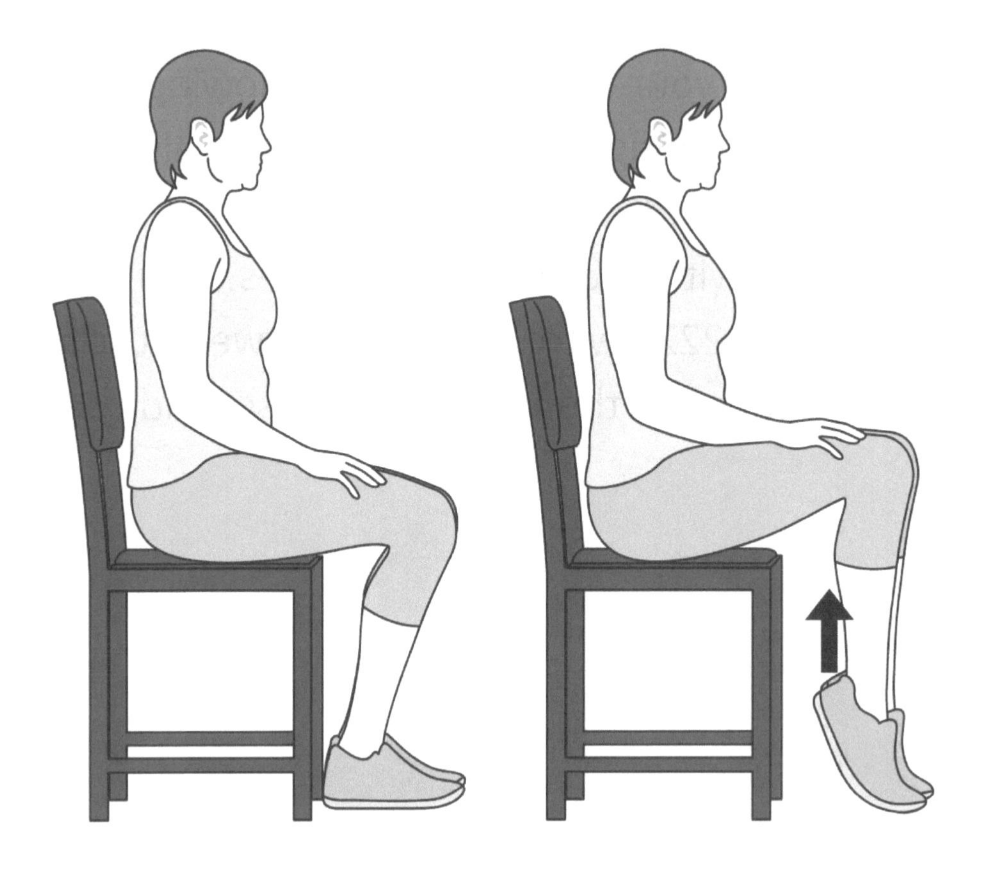

1. Begin by sitting upright in your chair with your shoulders down and back.

2. Place your feet directly under your knees.

3. Roll up to the balls of your feet so your knees raise. Raise it as high as you feel comfortable.

4. Roll back down so your heels rest back on the ground.

5. Repeat for 8 reps.

Target: Concentrate on the feeling of your calves tightening and moving smoothly between positions so your legs do not shake or bounce through the movement.

Making it easier: Use your hands to help guide and raise your knee.

Adding difficulty: Add resistance by pushing down on your raising knee with your hand as you lift, holding a weight over your knee, or looping a resistance band under the balls of your feet and wrapping it over your knees. You can also add a tempo of 3432, where it takes 3 seconds to raise, 4 seconds to hold, 3 seconds to lower, and 2 seconds to rest. If you still feel like you need to apply more resistance and your balance permits, you can also attempt rising on the balls of your feet while standing and holding the chair's backrest.

You now have a range of exercises that you can incorporate into your workout routine that will not only maintain and build lower-body strength but also help you maintain balance and stability.

Remember, you can choose which warm-up and cooldowns you want and focus on any particular combination of exercises.

Next up, we will look at shoulder and neck exercises that you can add to your training routine.

Your Chance to Inspire Others to Embrace Aging with Grace

At the outset of this book, I shared a core belief: Aging is not merely about the ticking of the clock but the quality of moments we choose to live. Each phase of life is an adventure, teeming with opportunities for body, mind, and spirit growth. I shared the illuminating encounter with Harriet, an 87-year-old beacon of positivity, and the transformative journey of Joan, who took her health and happiness into her own hands at 70. Their stories reveal a resounding truth: our golden years can be as fulfilling as any other chapter in our life, if not more.

But this realization doesn't come easily to all. Feelings of waning youth, physical limitations, and the shadows of missed opportunities can cloud one's perspective. Many face the risk of declining mobility and the weight of emotional and physical challenges. But, as we've explored together, there's a powerful remedy: staying active and embracing a proactive approach to well-being.

By now, you've dived deep into the potential benefits of exercise, not just as a physical tool but as a means to rejuvenate spirit and passion. As Joan's journey and countless others suggest, it's never too late to make positive change. And this is where you come in. Your experience with this book could serve as a beacon for countless others on a similar journey.

By leaving a review of this book on Amazon, you guide other seniors and their loved ones toward a path of health, vibrancy, and fulfillment.

Simply by sharing how these chair exercises have transformed your daily life and what newcomers can anticipate, you lay down stepping stones for others to walk a healthier, happier path.

Thank you for your support. As you continue to flourish in your journey of graceful aging, remember that sharing insights and stories is a beautiful way to leave a legacy and inspire others. Embrace, share, and thrive!

Scan the QR code below

Neck and Shoulder Exercises

> At the end of the day, your health is your responsibility.
>
> Jillian Michaels

I want you to have the ability to hold your head up high as we gracefully move through our older years. Please allow me this pun as we move into our neck and shoulder exercise section—I couldn't help myself.

As we age, our posture changes, and we may have spent a good portion of our years seated behind a chair which could have caused structural changes to our bodies: the most significant being our backs and necks.

According to Alverson (2021), the benefits of strengthening your neck include:

- improved posture
- improved breathing
- improved balance and coordination
- reduced risk of injury
- reduced neck and back pain
- reduced tension and stiffness

We carry a lot on our shoulders, and I mean that both literally and figuratively. Exercise can help you relax by releasing stress and strengthening your upper body with the following exercises.

According to Pike et al. (2022), as we age, we experience a loss in shoulder strength, specifically once we reach around age 60. For our independence, we must keep our shoulders healthy and functioning optimally. Healthy shoulders mean we can continue to drive a car, carry our groceries, pick up our grandchildren, or do housework. Keeping our strength in our neck and shoulders sets us up for more years of carefree living and continuing to do what we love and need to do.

Neck Stretches

You can use these static stretches during your warm-up or cooldown routine. You can also use them on rest days to keep you active and improve your flexibility and mobility.

Here are three of the most influential and popular upper-body stretches. Please remember that we never stretch through pain. If you feel any pain or discomfort, please release the stretch.

Seated Neck Release

1. Begin by sitting upright in your chair with your shoulder blades down and back.

2. Your feet should be flat on the floor.

3. Place your right hand on your right thigh.

4. Place your left hand on the top right side of your head.

5. Exhale and gently pull your head to the left.

6. Hold for 30 seconds and release. Breathe deeply and sink into the stretch as you inhale and exhale.

7. Repeat on the other side.

Clasping Neck Stretch

1. Begin by sitting upright in your chair with your shoulder blades down and back.

2. Your feet should be flat on the floor.

3. Inhale, interlace your fingers and place them behind your head.

4. Continue to sit up straight and press your body firmly into your seat while you press your hands towards your thighs. Deeply exhale as you do so.

5. Tuck your chin into your chest while you do this.

6. Hold for 30 seconds and release.

Eagle Arm Stretch

1. Begin by sitting upright in your chair with your shoulder blades down and back.

2. Your feet should be flat on the floor.

3. Lift your arms forward in line with your shoulders and your palms facing each other.

4. At your elbows, bend your arms up to the ceiling.
5. Cross your arms, placing your right elbow in the crook of your left elbow pit.
6. Rotate your wrists and clasp your hands together as best as possible.
7. Lift your arms in this configuration as high as you feel comfortable. You should feel the stretch in your shoulders and upper back.
8. Hold this stretch for 10-15 seconds while breathing deeply and relaxing into the stretch.
9. Release and relax the arms at your sides or in your lap.
10. Lift your arms forward in line with your shoulders and repeat the stretch with your left elbow in the crook of your right elbow pit this time.
11. Hold the stretch for 10-15 seconds, then release.

Neck Exercises

Neck Flexion

This exercise helps in relieving tension in the posterior neck muscles. Regular practice can aid in improving the range of motion in the neck and reducing stiffness.

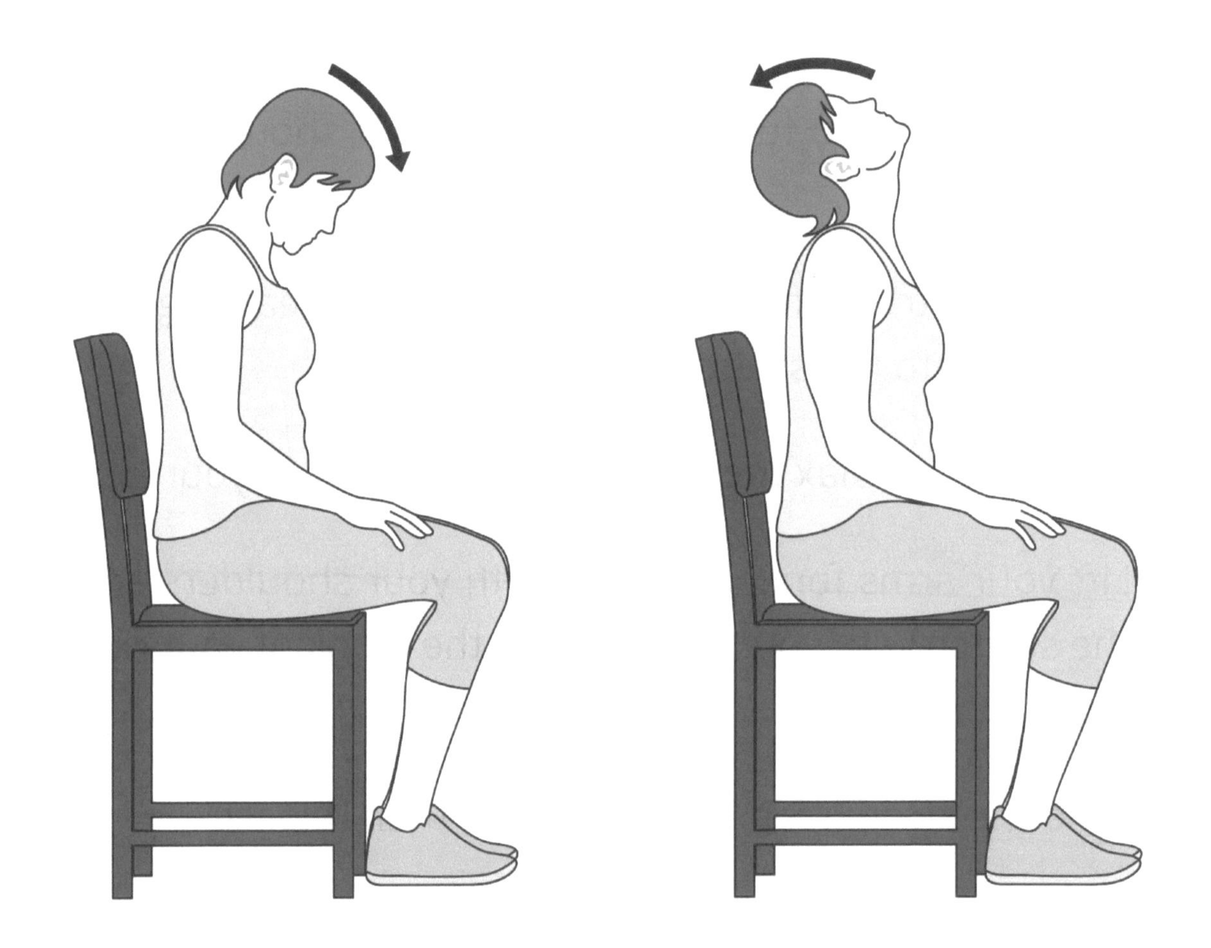

1. Begin by sitting upright in your chair with your shoulder blades down and back.

2. Your feet should be flat on the floor.

3. Inhale and look upwards and tilt your head as far back as comfortable.

4. Exhale and bring your chin down to your chest.
5. Repeat for 8 reps.

Target: We want to create a gentle stretch along the back and front of the neck while ensuring the spine remains in line, moving slowly during the movement and pausing at the top and bottom.

Making it easier: Take an extra moment in you feel slightly disorientated at any point before continuing the movement. Reduce the range of motion, only going as far as you feel comfortable.

Adding difficulty: Add a tempo of 4242 to establish a good rhythm of movement. You can use your hand to assist your head movement and deepen the stretch.

Neck Rotations

Regular neck rotations increase lateral neck flexibility. They are also essential for maintaining a healthy range of motion and reducing neck pain.

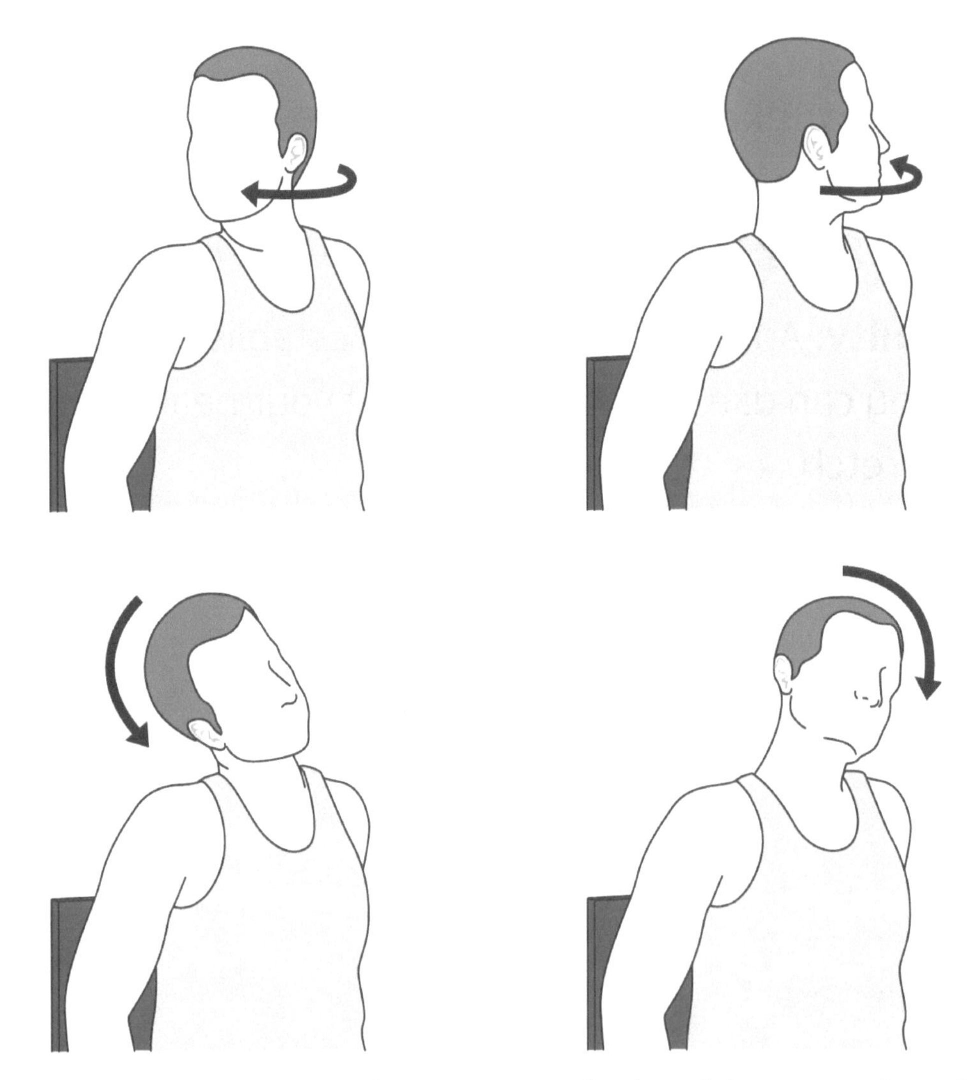

1. Begin by sitting upright in your chair with your shoulder blades down and back.

2. Your feet should be flat on the floor.

3. Exhale and gently turn your neck to look over your left shoulder. Go as far as you feel comfortable.

4. Inhale and return to the neutral position.
5. Exhale and gently turn your neck to look over your right shoulder. Go as far as you feel comfortable.
6. Repeat for 6 reps.
7. Inhale and return your head to the neutral position.
8. Exhale and gently tilt your left ear to your shoulder. Go as far as you feel comfortable.
9. Inhale and return to the neutral position.
10. Exhale and gently tilt your left ear to your shoulder. Go as far as you feel comfortable.
11. Inhale and return to the neutral position.
12. Repeat for 6 reps.

Target: We want to rotate and tilt our heads smoothly between positions feeling a gentle stretch in the sides of our neck while keeping the shoulder stationary.

Making it easier: Take an extra moment in you feel slightly disorientated at any point before continuing the movement. Reduce the range of motion, only going as far as you feel comfortable.

Adding difficulty: Add a tempo of 4242 to establish a good rhythm of movement. You can use your hand to assist your head movement and deepen the stretch.

Levator Scapulae

This exercise benefits those experiencing tightness or discomfort in the neck and upper shoulders. It targets the muscle that runs from the cervical spine to the shoulder blades, ensuring a reduction in tension and improved posture.

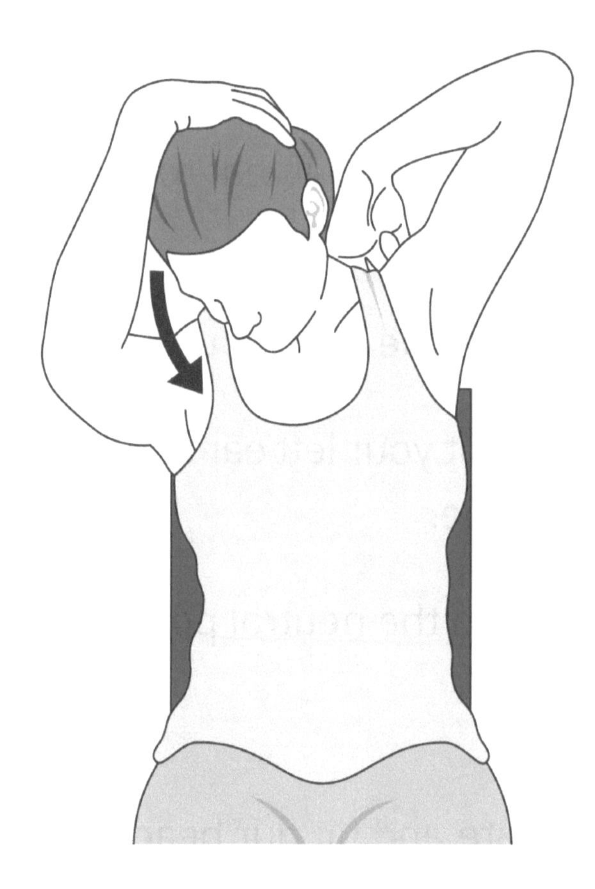

1. Begin by sitting upright in your chair with your shoulder blades down and back.

2. Your feet should be flat on the floor.

3. Inhale and place your right hand behind your back on your right shoulder blade.

4. Exhale, turn your head to the left at about a 45° angle and look down at your right knee. Use your left hand to gently pull your

head lower toward your knee to increase the stretch. Breathe in and out as you stretch and sink deeper into the hold.

5. You should feel a stretch behind the right side of your neck.
6. Hold for 20 seconds.
7. Return to a neutral position and repeat on the other side.

Target: We want to focus on the muscle that runs from the cervical spine down to the shoulder blades, alleviating tension in the neck and upper shoulders.

Making it easier: Do not use your hand to pull the head down; rely solely on the head's weight for the stretch.

Adding difficulty: Increase the hold time or gently apply more pressure to deepen the stretch with your hand.

Shoulder Exercises

Shoulder Rolls

Shoulder rolls are excellent for increasing circulation to the shoulder joints, relieving tension, and promoting fluid motion. Regular shoulder rolls can help prevent stiffness and improve upper back posture.

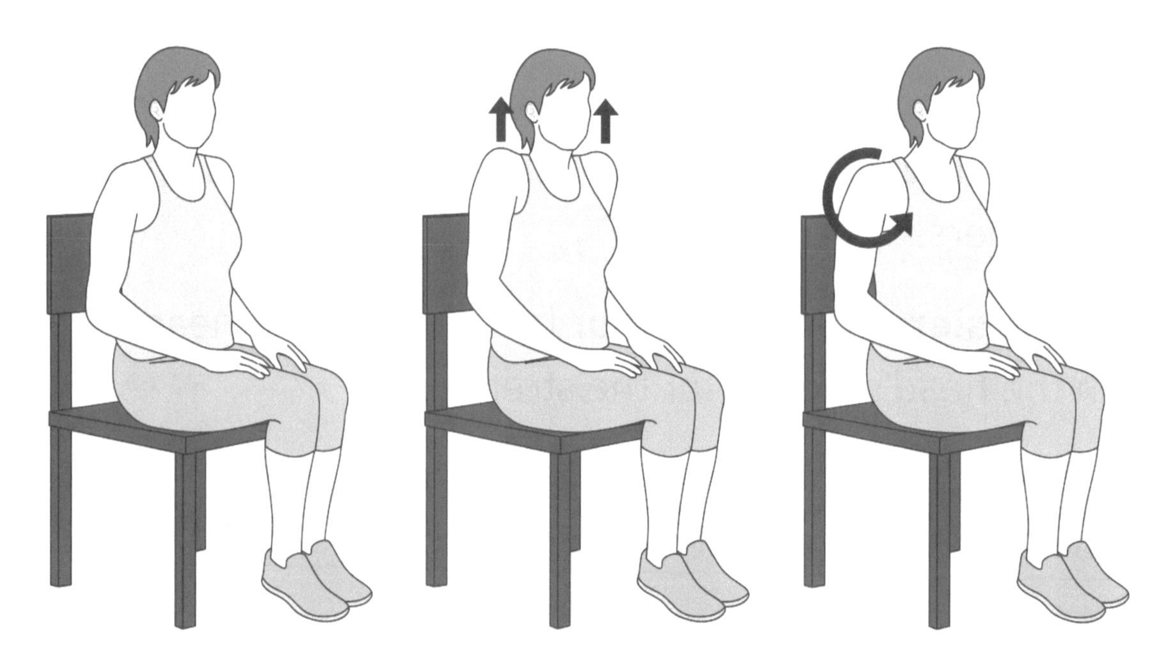

1. Begin by sitting upright in your chair with your shoulder blades down and back.

2. Your feet should be flat on the floor.

3. Place your palms on your thighs.

4. Inhale and shrug your shoulders up towards your ears and roll them back toward the backrest of your chair. Concentrate on squeezing your shoulder blades together as you do so.

5. As you come back down, push them forward and back up to the top of the shrug to complete the circle.

6. Repeat for the recommended amount of repetitions.
7. Return to neutral.
8. Inhale and shrug your shoulders up towards your ears. Roll them forward.
9. As you come back down, push them backward, concentrating on squeezing your shoulder blades together and completing the circle.
10. Repeat for 8 reps.

Target: We want to fully explore our range of motion, ensuring we raise our shrug as high as possible, pinching the shoulder blades together as we reach the back, dropping our shoulders at the bottom, and curling our shoulders forward.

Making it easier: Reduce the range of motion by performing a smaller roll.

Adding difficulty: Flex your forearms out when you roll to the back and rotate your forearms when you roll forward. Increase the reps or use a resistance band between your hands with the added forearm movement.

Bicep Curl Into Shoulder Press

This compound exercise aims to strengthen the biceps and deltoid muscles simultaneously. Integrating two movements also promotes upper-body coordination and ensures balanced muscle development.

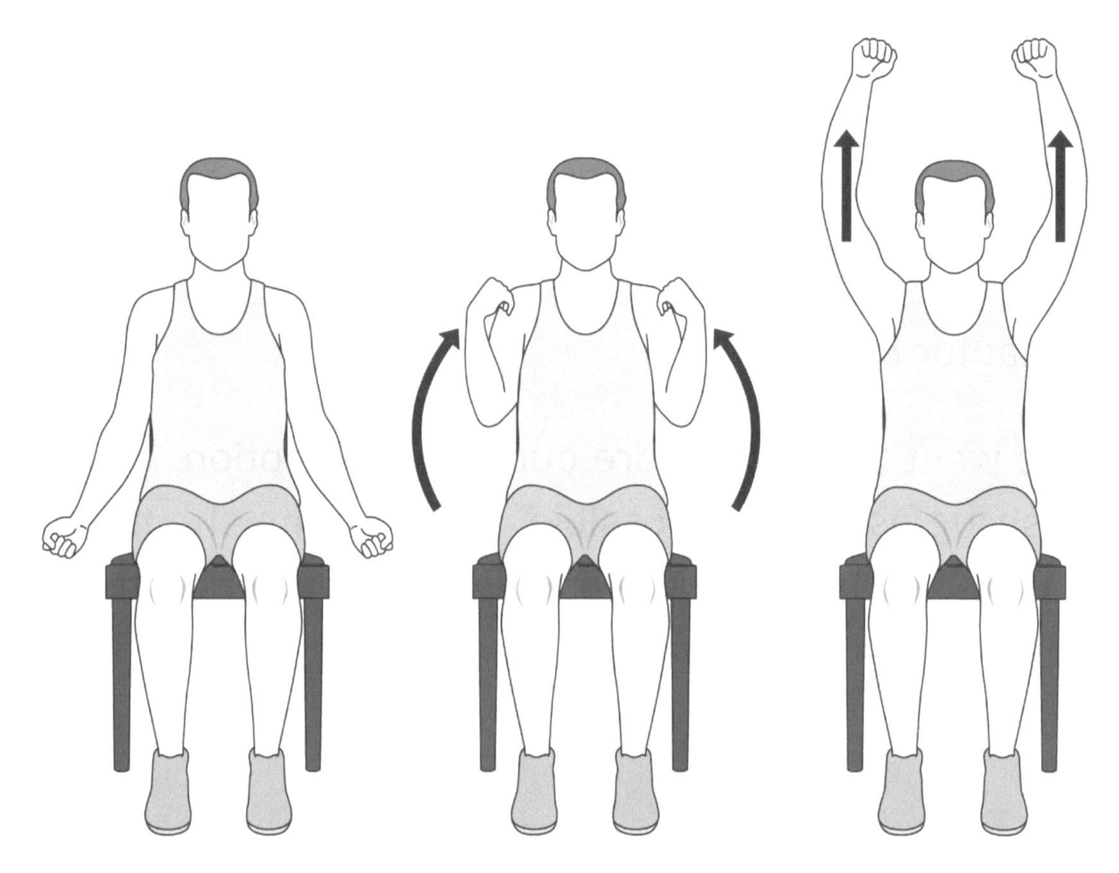

1. Begin by sitting upright in your chair with your shoulder blades down and back.

2. Your feet should be flat on the floor.

3. Inhale and bring your arms to the side with your palms facing outwards.

4. Curl your arms from the elbow all the way to your shoulders. Once your fingers touch your shoulders, breathe out, straighten, and press your hands up overhead with your arms should be next to your ears and in line with your shoulders.

5. Lower your hands to touch your shoulders and uncurl them back into their straight starting position.

6. Repeat for 8 reps.

Target: We want to move smoothly with control through the transition between curls up through the shoulder press and back down again.

Making it easier: Limit your range of motion by not extending your arms fully or reducing the volume of reps.

Adding difficulty: Add weights or a resistance band with the ends in your hands and the middle either under your thighs or securely under your feet so it will not slip out. Increase the volume of reps or a tempo of 6362.

Shoulder Flexions

Shoulder flexions focus on enhancing the frontal range of motion in the shoulders. Regularly practicing this exercise can assist in maintaining healthy shoulder joints, improving posture, and reducing the risk of shoulder-related issues.

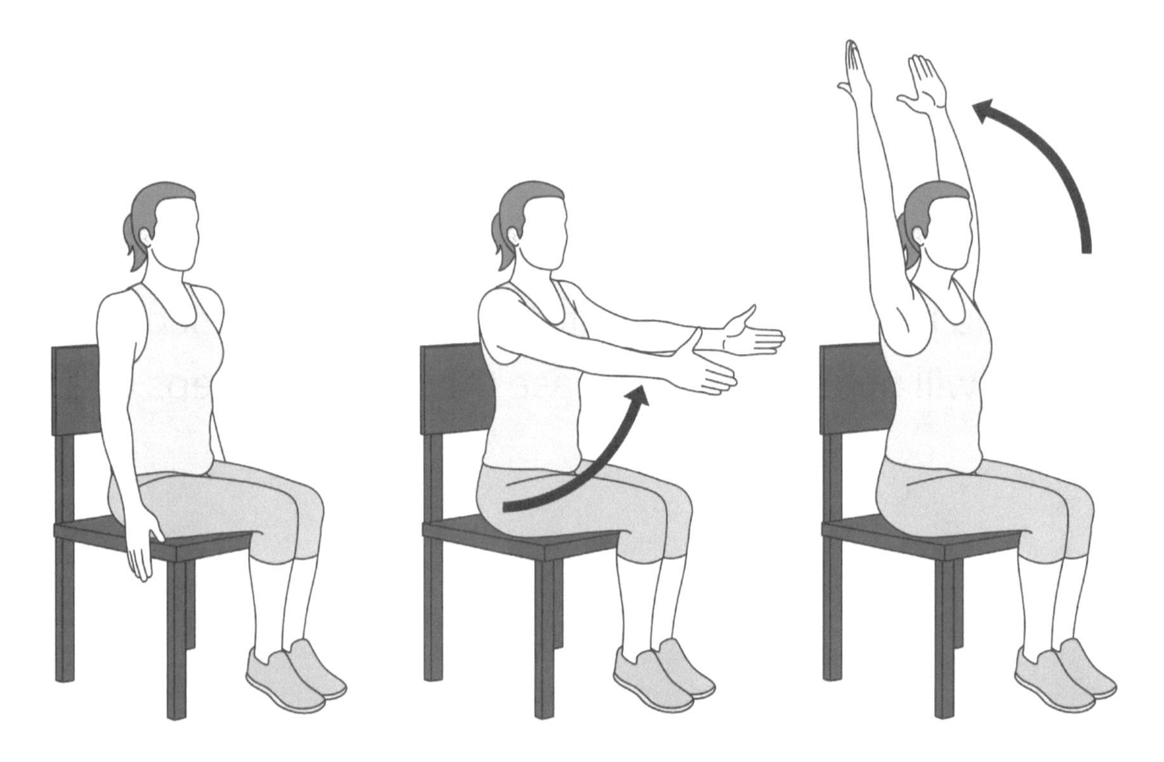

1. Begin by sitting upright in your chair with your shoulder blades down and back.
2. Your feet should be flat on the floor.
3. Let your arms hang at your side with your thumbs facing forward.
4. Keeping your arms straight, inhale and lift them as high as possible to get them overhead and in line with your ears.
5. Slowly bring them down to your sides.

6. Repeat for 8 reps.

Target: We want to keep our backs and arms straight, slowly moving them in a gentle arc from the bottom of the position to over our heads and back.

Making it easier: Reduce the range of motion, lifting your arms only to shoulder height or slightly above before bringing them back down.

Adding difficulty: Add weights or a resistance band with the ends in your hands and the middle under your feet so it will not slip out. You can also add a tempo of 5362 or increase the volume of reps.

Shoulder Circles

Shoulder circles can aid in enhancing the overall mobility of the shoulder joints. They help in loosening tight muscles around the shoulder girdle to increase flexibility.

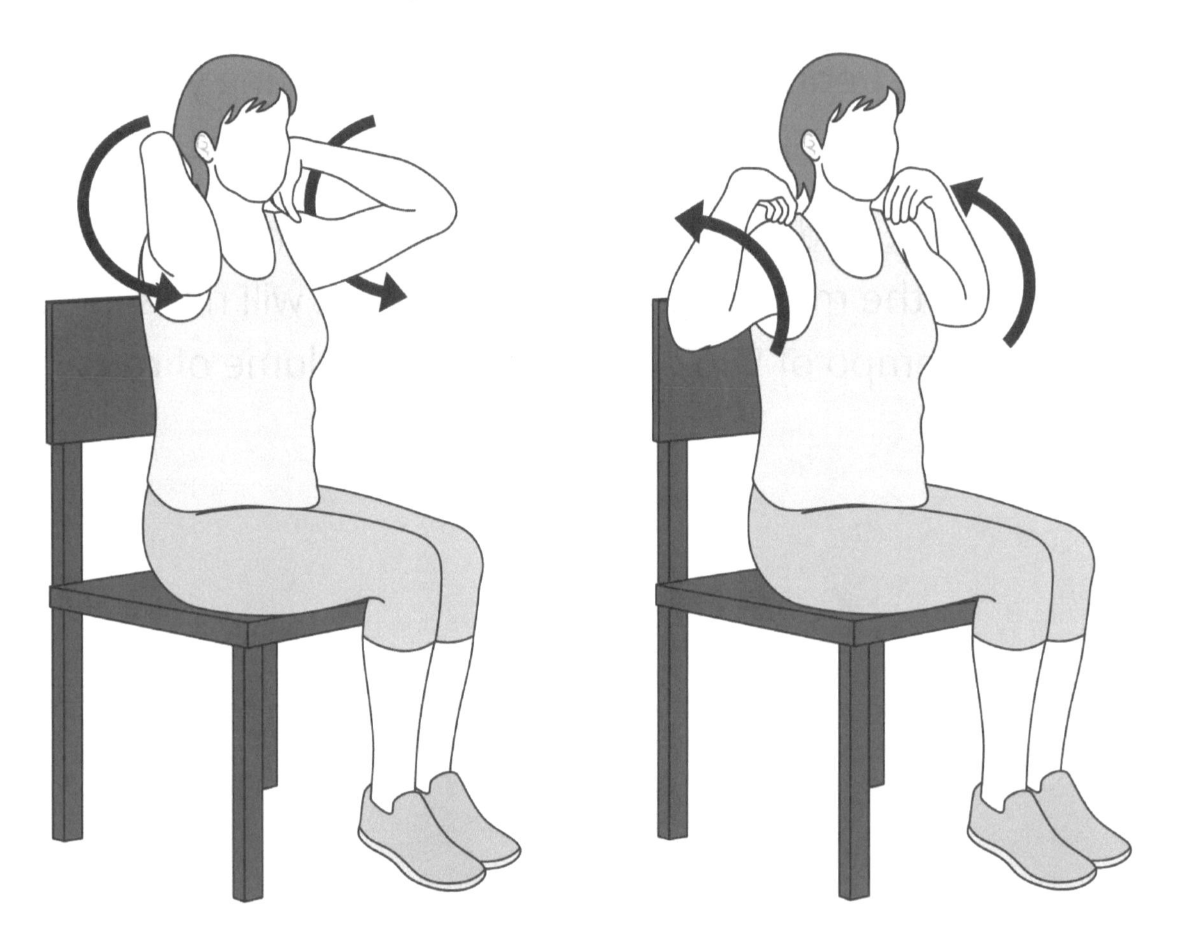

1. Begin by sitting upright in your chair with your shoulder blades down and back.
2. Your feet should be flat on the floor.
3. Place your fingertips on your shoulders.
4. Moving from your shoulders but leading with your elbow, rotate your arms backward in a wide circle.
5. Repeat for 8 reps.

6. Moving from your shoulders but leading with your elbow, rotate your arms forward in a wide circle.

7. Repeat for 8 reps.

Target: We want to focus on moving the elbows out and generating smooth circles by engaging the muscles around the shoulder joint.

Making it easier: Decrease the size of the circles. Instead of a full, broad rotation, focus on smaller, controlled circles.

Adding difficulty: Slow down the movement significantly, ensuring that every rotation part is controlled and deliberate.

Great work. We now have another couple of workouts we can rotate through as we build our exercise program. In the next chapter, we will stick to the upper body and work on our upper- and lower-back muscles. These movements are also movements that will help us retain good posture.

Upper and Lower Back Exercises

> Those who think they have no time for bodily exercise will sooner or later have to find time for illness.
>
> Edward Stanley

Not only will these exercises make you stronger, but they can also improve your posture. We need to maintain good posture as it helps keep our spines healthy.

Long hours spent driving, slumped on a couch, hovering over a cell phone, or sleeping in strange positions can result in lower back pain and tension. Our poor posture leads to compromised mechanics in our movements, affecting us persistently throughout the day.

These exercises can be a great source of pain relief. Still, they can also help counteract poor posture and ensure you keep yourself well while participating in your daily activities.

Upper and Lower Back Stretches

Goddess With a Twist

1. Begin by sitting upright towards the front of your chair with your shoulders down and back.

2. As you breathe in, open your legs wide and point your toes

outwards.

3. Exhale and place your right arm inside your right leg with your palm facing forwards.
4. Raise your left arm towards the ceiling and shift your gaze upward to look at your left palm.
5. Hold this position for five deep breaths.
6. Return to a neutral position.
7. Repeat on the other side.

Seated Rotation

1. Begin by sitting upright towards the front of your chair with your shoulders down and back.
2. As you breathe in, cross your arms over your chest.
3. Leading with your arms, exhale and rotate your torso to the left as far as you feel comfortable.
4. Hold for two to three deep breaths.
5. Exhale and rotate your torso to the right as far as you feel comfortable.
6. Hold for two to three deep breaths.
7. Repeat for 6 reps on both sides.

Lower Back Exercises

Seated Cat-Cow

This exercise promotes movement through the entire length of your spine, relieving stiffness and engaging your core for stability.

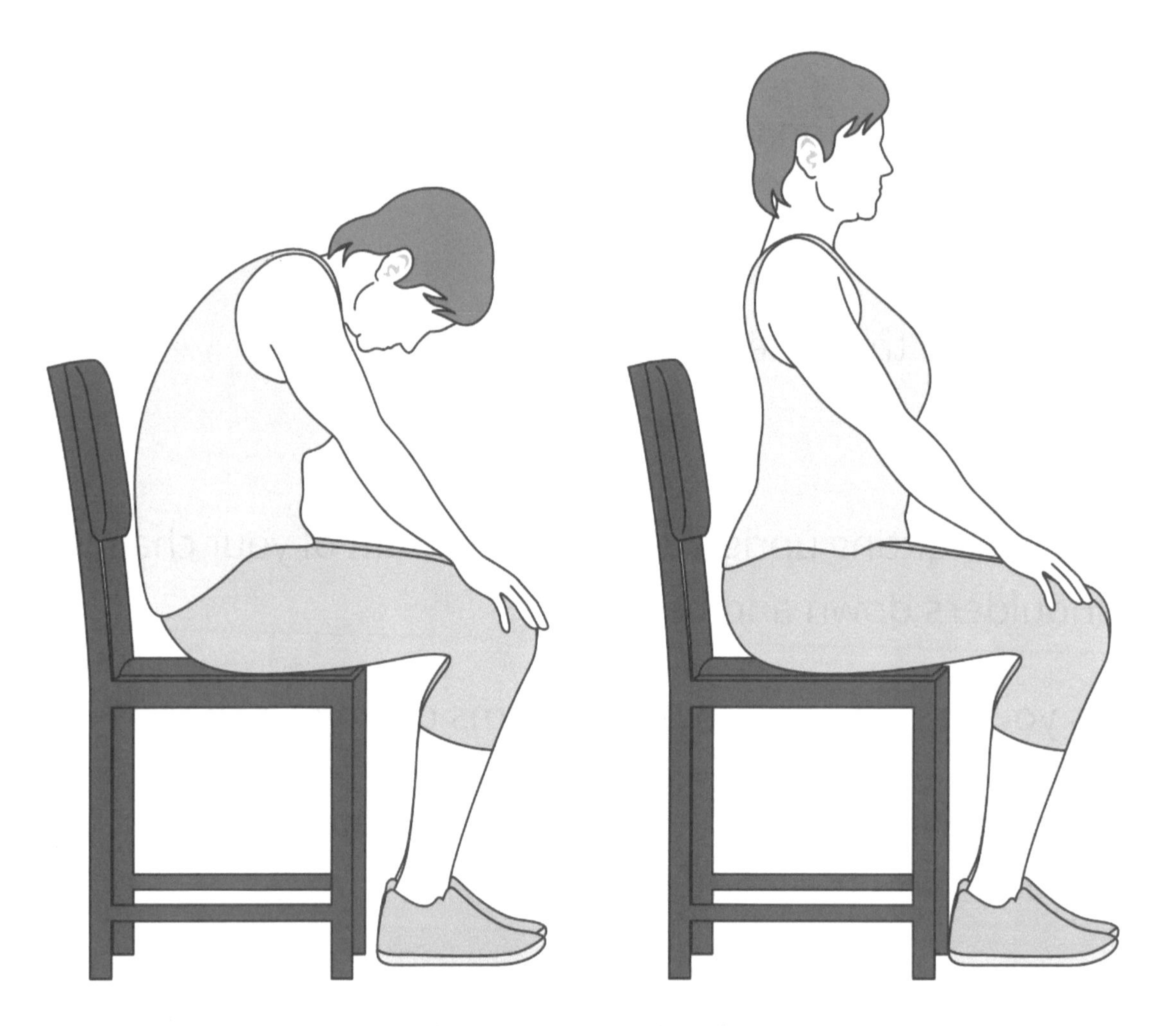

1. Begin by sitting upright towards the front of your chair with your shoulders down and back.

2. Place both feet underneath your knees, planting them firmly on the floor.

3. Place your hands on your thighs for stability and Inhale.

4. Exhale and round your spine forward vertebra by vertebra while

you slide your hands forward for balance to your knees.

5. Inhale and straighten your spine as you come up and continue moving backward as you arch your spine and roll your shoulders back, sliding your hands back to the resting position.

6. Repeat for 8 reps.

Target: We want to use smooth, controlled movement between the arching and rounding our backs, breathing between the positions' top and bottom.

Making it easier: Limit your range of motion, and take longer breaks if the movement makes you feel light-headed.

Adding difficulty: Add a tempo of 5353 or add more reps. You can also place your hand behind your head, ensuring you are not pulling on your neck or head.

Gentle Twist

This is a gentle exercise that works to relieve back tension and improve mobility.

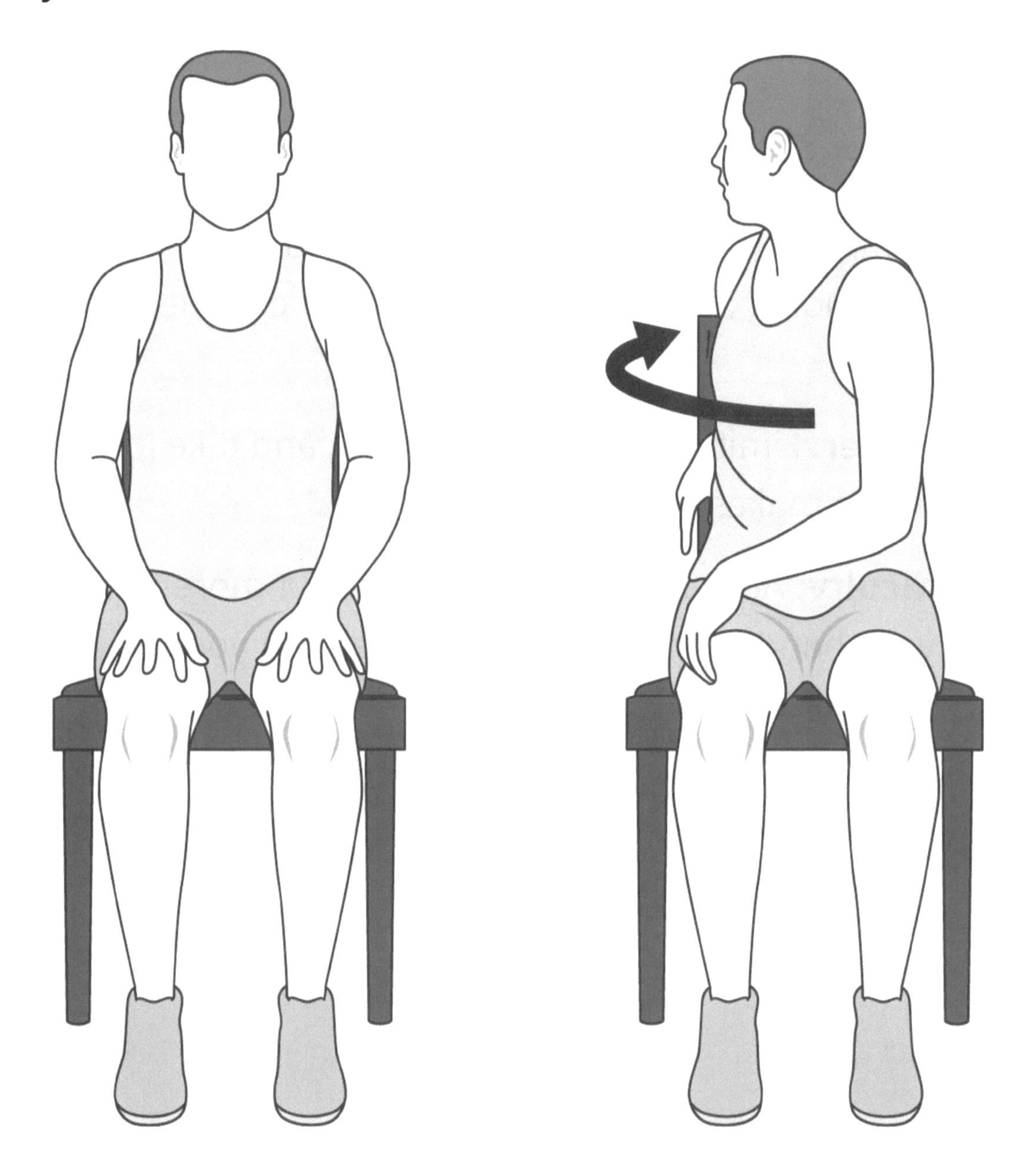

1. Begin by sitting upright towards the front of your chair with your shoulders down and back.

2. Place both feet underneath your knees, firmly planting them on the floor.

3. Inhale, place your left hand on your right knee, rotate your upper body reach, and grab the chair's backrest with your right hand.
4. Exhale breathing deeper into the stretch.
5. Inhale, moving slowly to the other side.
6. Exhale, placing your right hand on your left knee rotating and grabbing the chair's backrest with your left hand.
7. Repeat on both sides for 6 reps.

Target: We want to lead with our head rotating the rest of our body with it.

Making it easier: Limit your range of movement.

Adding difficulty: Hold the position for longer, deepening the stretch as you breathe in and out.

Lumbar Extension

This exercise is a great way to reduce lower back strains and pain by stretching the lower back into a more natural curved posture.

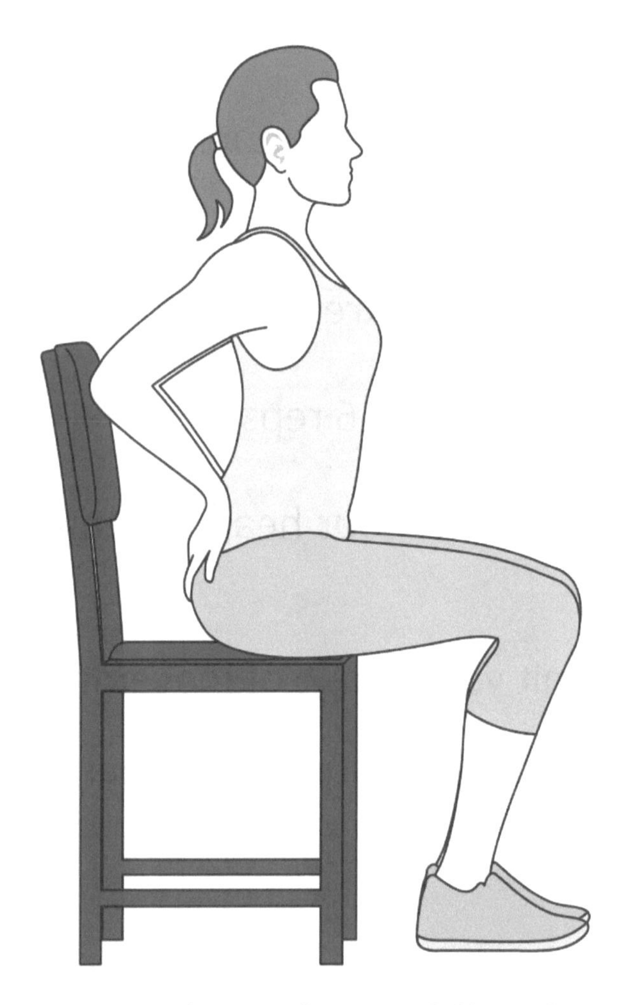

1. Begin by sitting upright in the middle of your chair with your shoulders down and back.

2. Place both feet underneath your knees, firmly planting them on the floor.

3. Inhale and place your hands on the small of your back.

4. As you breathe out, lean backward into your hands and extend into your lower back.

5. Hold for five deep breaths. Sink into the movement as you breathe in and out.

Target: We want to keep a neutral spine, not straining or twisting our backs in either direction.

Making it easier: Lean your elbows back into the chair's backrest to aid in balance and reduce the range of movement.

Adding difficulty: Add a tempo of 3532 or hold a weight at your chest.

Lumbar Side Flexion

This exercise strengthens your obliques and quadratus lumborum, the muscles that run on your sides and back below your rib cage. It also helps stabilize your back, aiding in your balance and mobility.

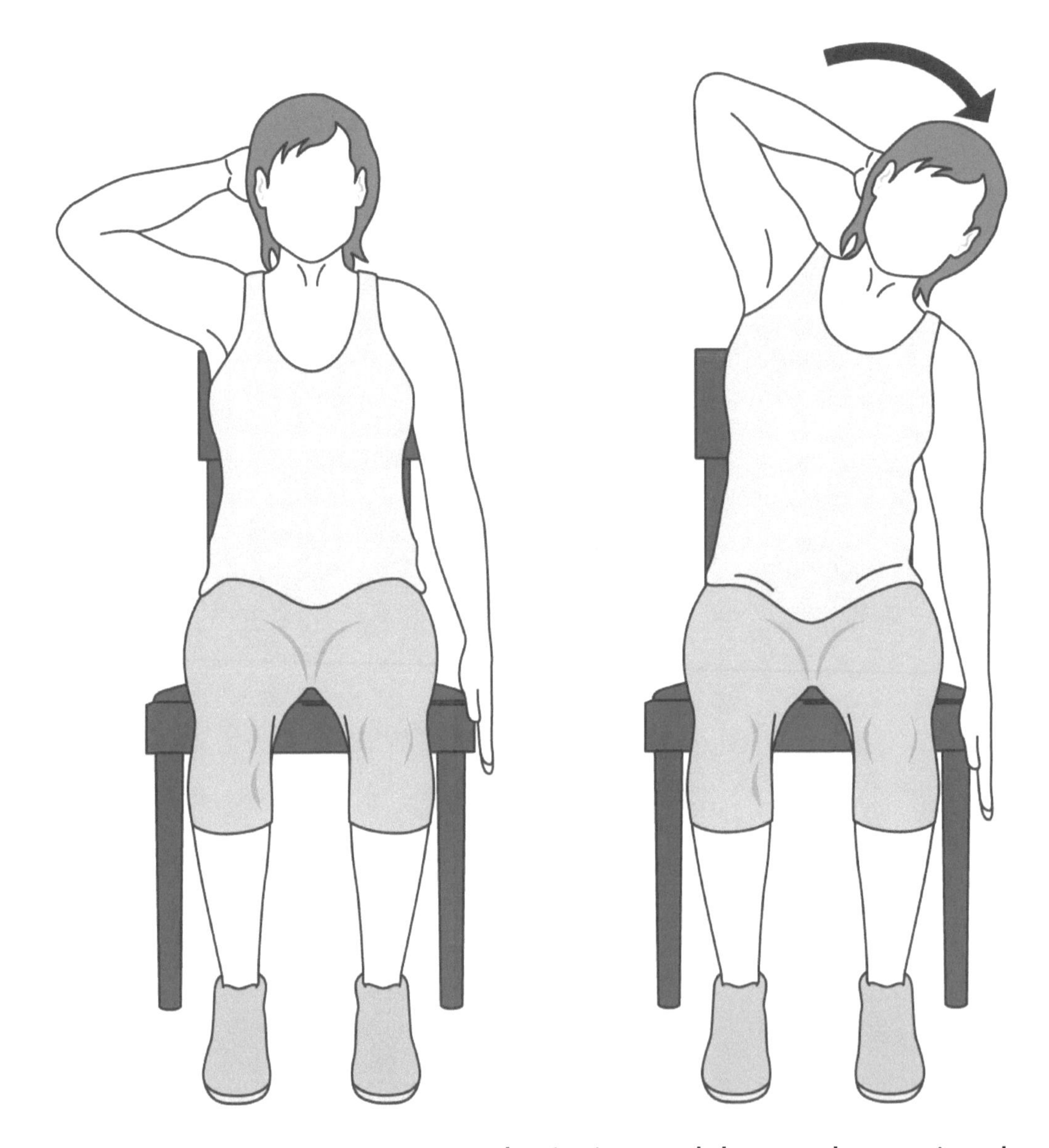

Safety Moment: Ensure your chair is stable and not in danger of tipping with your weight for this exercise.

1. Begin by sitting upright in your chair with your shoulders down and back.
2. Place both feet underneath your knees, firmly planting them on

the floor.

3. Inhale and place your right hand behind your head with your left hand down at your side.

4. Exhale and lower your left arm toward the ground while raising your right elbow toward the ceiling. Go as far as you feel comfortable.

5. Repeat for 5 reps.

6. Inhale and place your left hand behind your head with your right hand down at your side.

7. Exhale and lower your right arm toward the ground while raising your left elbow toward the ceiling. Go as far as you feel comfortable.

8. Repeat for 8 reps on each side.

Target: We want to bend only between the bottom of our ribs and hip, feeling the stretch on our opposite side.

Making it easier: Limit your range of motion to where you feel comfortable. Place your chair near a wall for support as you lean against it, or spread your feet wider to aid in balance.

Adding difficulty: You can add a tempo of 3432 or increase the volume of reps. Additionally, you could hold a dumbbell weight in hand at your side or place a resistance band under your right foot, ensuring it will not slip out when you exercise, and hold the other end with your right hand as you bend to your left side.

Seated Roll Down

This exercise articulates the spine slowly to improve mobility and flexibility for your entire spinal column. It also strengthens your core muscles as you control the speed of your movement.

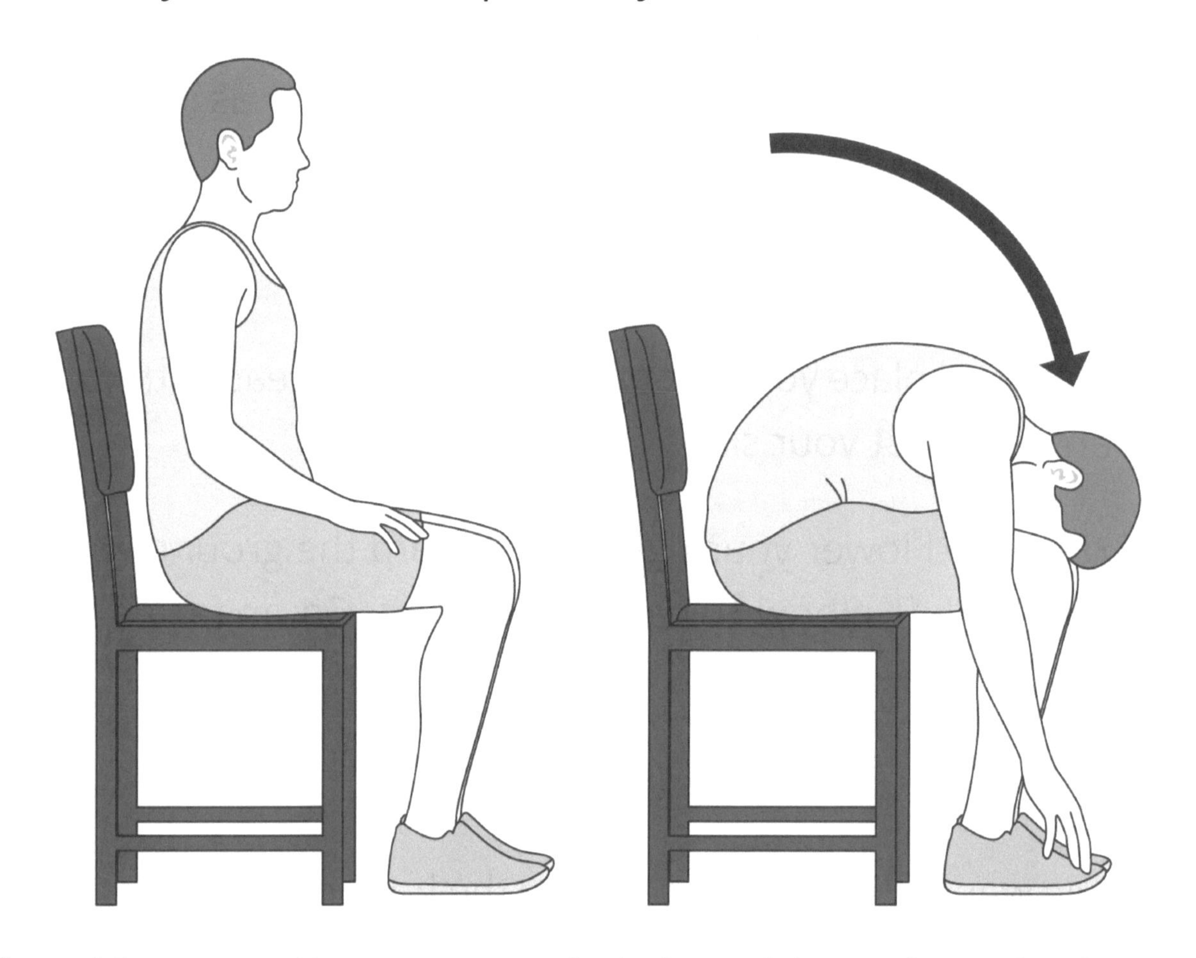

Safety Moment: Ensure your chair is stable and not in danger of tipping forward with your weight for this exercise.

1. Begin by sitting upright towards the front of your chair with your shoulders down and back.

2. Place both feet underneath your knees, firmly planting them on the floor.

3. Place your hands on your thighs and Inhale.

4. Exhale and slide your hands to your knees and down your legs to the floor or as far as you feel comfortable, curving your back forward vertebra by vertebra.

5. Inhale and slowly roll yourself vertebra by vertebra back to the starting position while you slide your hands back up your legs to your knees, then back to your thighs.

6. Repeat for 6 reps.

Target: We want to concentrate on moving slowly, one vertebra at a time, as we bend down and back up.

Making it easier: Use your hands to guide and support your upper body weight as you move throughout the exercise. Reduce your range of motion by only going as far as you feel comfortable, slowly adding more range as you build confidence, strength, and flexibility.

Adding difficulty: Try extending your legs to change the body angle to engage more of your core while maintaining your balance and control. Add a tempo of 6262, or limit how much you rely on your hands on your legs.

Thoracic Rotation

This exercise improves mobility and flexibility of the upper back, where your ribcage attaches to your spine. As such, it not only alleviates back pain but also boosts the mobility of your ribcage and enhances lung expansion, leading to better breathing.

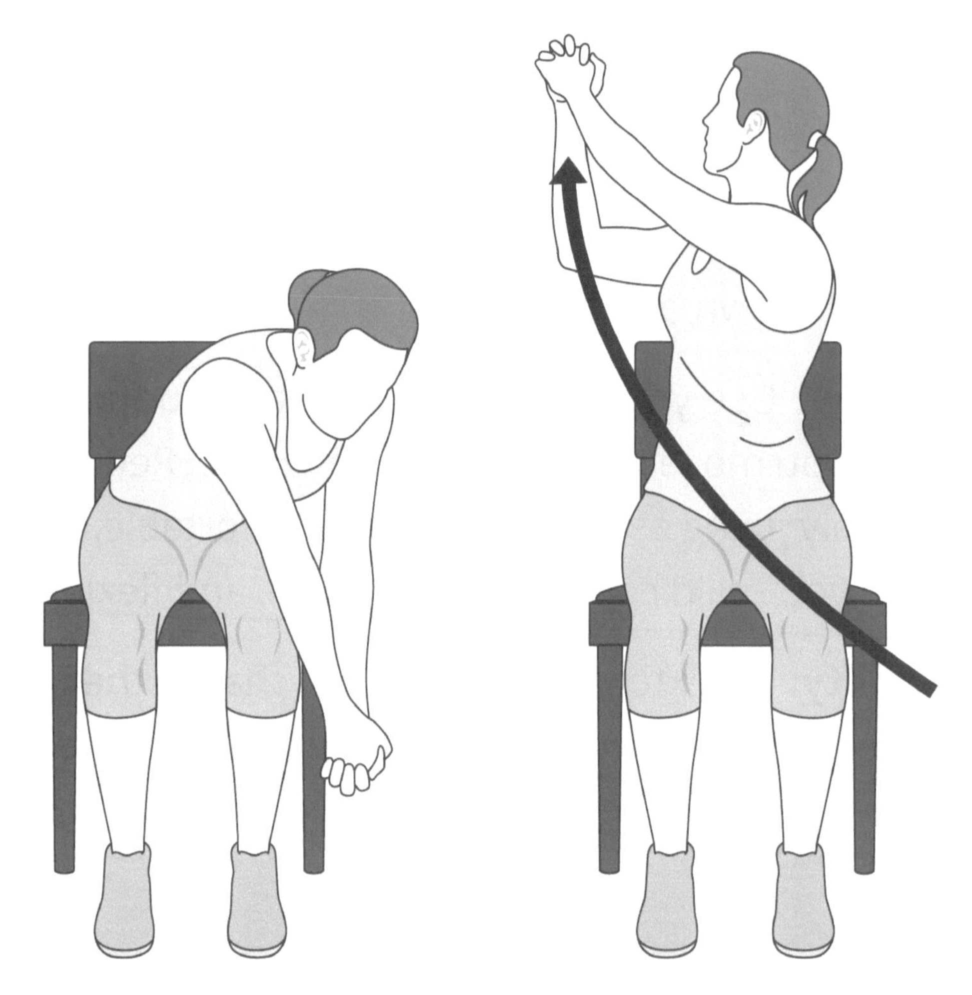

Safety Moment: Ensure your chair is stable and not in danger of tipping forward with your weight.

1. Begin by sitting upright towards the front of your chair with your shoulders down and back.

2. Place both feet underneath your knees, firmly planting them on the floor.

3. Inhale and clasp your hands together with your fingers interwoven in front of you.

4. Exhale and lower your clasped hands to the outside of your left lower leg so your right elbow is next to your left knee or as far as you feel comfortable.

5. Inhale and move your clasped hands in a gentle arc diagonally up to above your right shoulder and push your hands up as far as you feel comfortable.

6. Exhale and lower your clasped hands diagonally back down next to your left leg again.

7. Repeat the left-to-right sequence for 6 reps,

8. Repeat the sequence on the opposite side, starting with your clasped hands next to your right calf, moving diagonally over your left shoulder and back again.

9. Repeat the right-to-left sequence for 6 reps.

Target: We want to keep our head and eyes focused on our clasped hands as we rotate our back and shoulders through the movement.

Making it easier: Reduce the reps and only take the movement as far as you feel comfortable. You can also pull your clasped hands toward the bottom of your ribcage before raising them above the opposite shoulder.

Adding difficulty: Adding a tempo of 5452 or holding a dumbbell weight between your clasped hands and changing the volume of reps.

90° Lateral Stretch

This exercise may seem daunting at first, but it is an excellent way to reduce tension and stress build-up in your shoulders and back. It also helps improve mobility and flexibility from your arms all the way down to your calves. As you hold the stretch, you are also strengthening your back and core muscles.

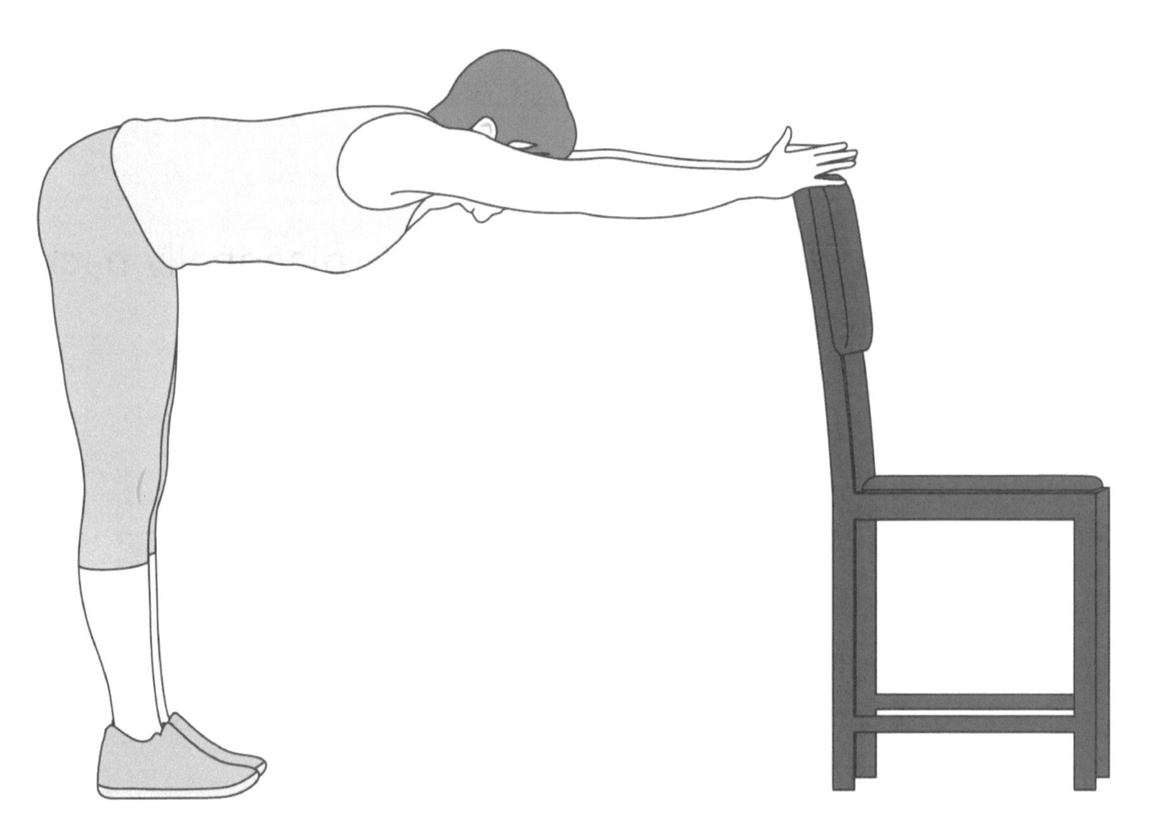

Safety Moment: Ensure your chair is stable and does not move away from you when you rest your hands during this exercise.

1. Begin by standing behind your chair with your feet shoulder-width apart and underneath your hips.

2. Inhale and raise your arms straight up above your head.

3. Exhale and bend forward at the hips, placing your hands on the chair's backrest.

4. Your arms should be straight in line with your shoulder and back, creating a 90-degree angle at your hips.

5. Focus on stretching your arms out, shoulders down, and lengthen your spine as you breathe in and out.

6. Hold for 15 seconds.

7. Step forward while holding the chair's backrest as you stand up and return to your normal posture.

Target: We want to focus on lengthening the spine while we are at 90 degrees with our hips, reaching out and forward with our hands to decompress the spine.

Making it easier: Reduce the time you hold the stretch. Keep your knees slightly bent if you feel discomfort in your hamstrings. You can also set up your chair near a wall that you can lean against for added stability until you can maintain your balance.

Adding difficulty: Increase the time you hold the pose and try over time to keep your legs straight.

Now that we have great exercises for improving our back posture and mobility in our repertoire, let us transition to improving our arms, wrists, and hands in the next chapter.

Arm, Wrist and Hand Exercises

> The last three or four reps is what makes the muscle grow. This area of pain divides the champion from someone else ho is not a champion.
>
> Arnold Schwarzenegger

Handstands, cartwheels, picking up and rocking babies, planting in our gardens, and putting away cans of beans—the mundane can seem unimportant until faced with it being taken from us. Out of all the benefits of being strong, we barely mention that one of the perks and benefits is that it just feels good to be capable.

Think about all the little things we need upper body strength for, such as holding, grasping, pulling, opening, or clenching. You need to be able to write and perform other small fine-motor-skilled based tasks. A tricep workout might not mean much, but it does mean you can continue to crochet that winter blanket with ease.

Arm Stretches

Prayer Stretch

1. Begin by sitting upright towards the front of your chair with your shoulders down and back. Ensure your chair is stable and not in danger of tipping forward with your weight.

2. Place both feet underneath your knees, firmly planting them on the floor.

3. Inhale and bring your palms together in front of your chest.

4. As you slowly breathe out, lower your elbow and raise your hands, keeping your palms together.

5. Gently press into your hands, holding this for three to five seconds.

6. Release and repeat 3 reps.

Overhead Reach

1. Begin by sitting upright in your chair with your shoulders down and back.

2. Place both feet underneath your knees, firmly planting them on the floor.

3. Inhale and interlock your fingers together in front of you.

4. Exhale and raise your arms overhead, turning your palms to face the ceiling as you do so.

5. Press up as high as you can.

6. Hold this position for five deep breaths.

7. Release and repeat for 3 reps.

Upper and Lower Arm Exercises

You can perform these exercises with any weights or resistance bands you wish or without. Remember, it is not how much weight or resistance you can lift or move but about the quality of movement and proper muscle engagement. Always opt for a lighter resistance or weight to ensure good form before progressing to harder difficulty.

Tricep Kickbacks

This exercise increases strength in the upper arm, mobility in the elbow, stability, and balance as you move the weight through the exercise.

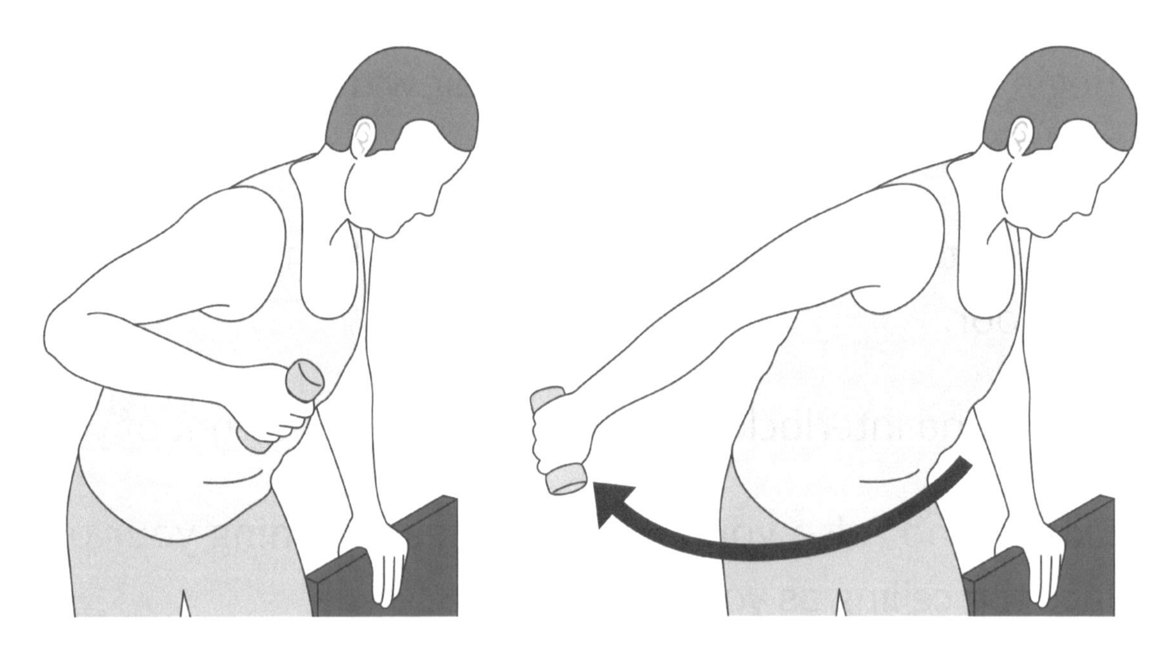

1. Beginning by standing upright behind your chair with your shoulders down and back.
2. Your feet should be hip-width apart.
3. Bend from your hips and hold onto the back of your chair.
4. Let your left arm hang to your side, holding your weight, and

your right arm remain on your chair for support.

5. Breathe in and lift your weight to the front of your shoulder, keeping your arm close to your body.

6. Exhale and lower the weight down and backward, straightening your arm out behind your back.

7. Repeat for 8 reps.

8. Switch sides and perform 8 reps.

Target: We want to descend the weight down and behind us slowly in a gentle arc and then pull back slowly to the shoulder again.

Making it easier: This exercise can also be done while sitting by resting your opposite arm across your lower thighs. Reduce or forget the weights, decrease the volume of reps, or reduce the range of motion by how far you extend your arm back.

Adding difficulty: Add a tempo of 3242, increase the volume of reps, or increase the weight resistance.

Elbow Side Extensions

This exercise helps strengthen your shoulders and arms for pulling, pushing, or reaching sideways for objects away from the body, whether putting on a coat, holding the steering wheel while driving, opening doors, reaching in the cupboard, or combing your hair. All of these daily tasks become easier.

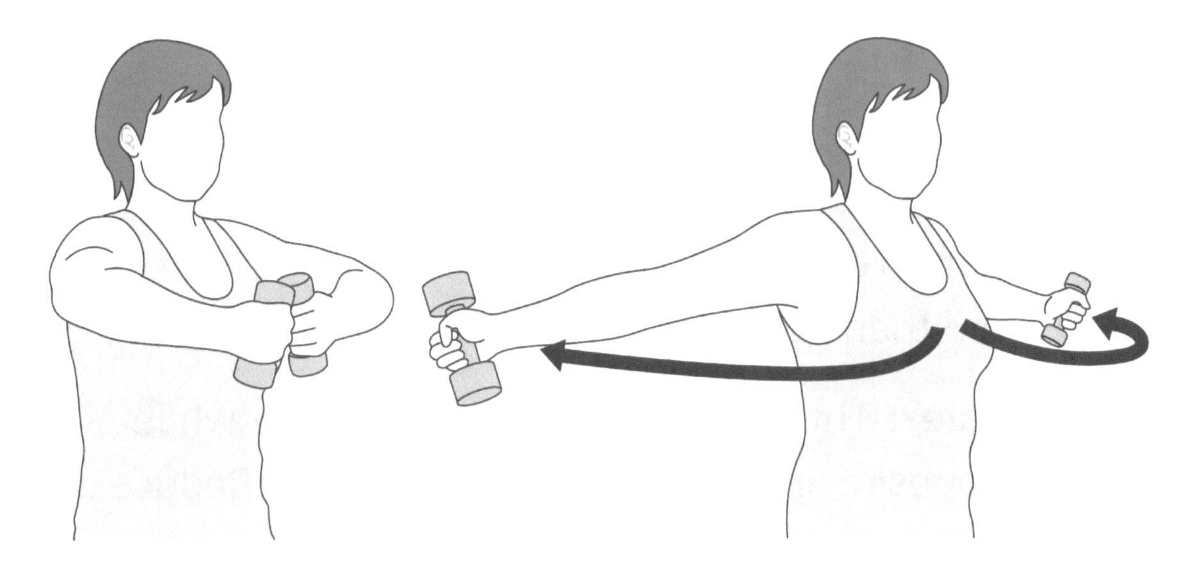

1. Begin by sitting upright in your chair with your shoulders down and back.

2. Place both feet underneath your knees, firmly planting them on the floor.

3. Inhale and hold your weights in your hand, bringing them together at your chest to touch each other.

4. Keep your shoulder blades down and back and your chest upright.

5. As you exhale, straighten your arms out to the side in line with your shoulders.

6. Inhale and bring them back to the center of your chest.

7. Repeat for 8 reps.

Target: We want to keep our arms up at the same plane as our shoulders and not let them droop. When our arms are fully open, we want to focus on pinching our shoulder blades together. The motion should be fluid as we open our arms wide and close them to our chest.

Making it easier: Feel free to do this exercise without the weights or reduce the volume of reps. You can also reduce the movement by leaving your elbows slightly bent in the open position.

Adding difficulty: Try adding a tempo of 3232 or increasing the weight or volume of reps. Alternatively, you can hold the ends of a resistance band in each hand.

Tricep Lifts

This exercise strengthens our arms' ability to push or lower ourselves into or out of a sitting position. It enables us to control our rise and descent instead of just dropping into a chair or using our leaning momentum until we get our weight over our feet.

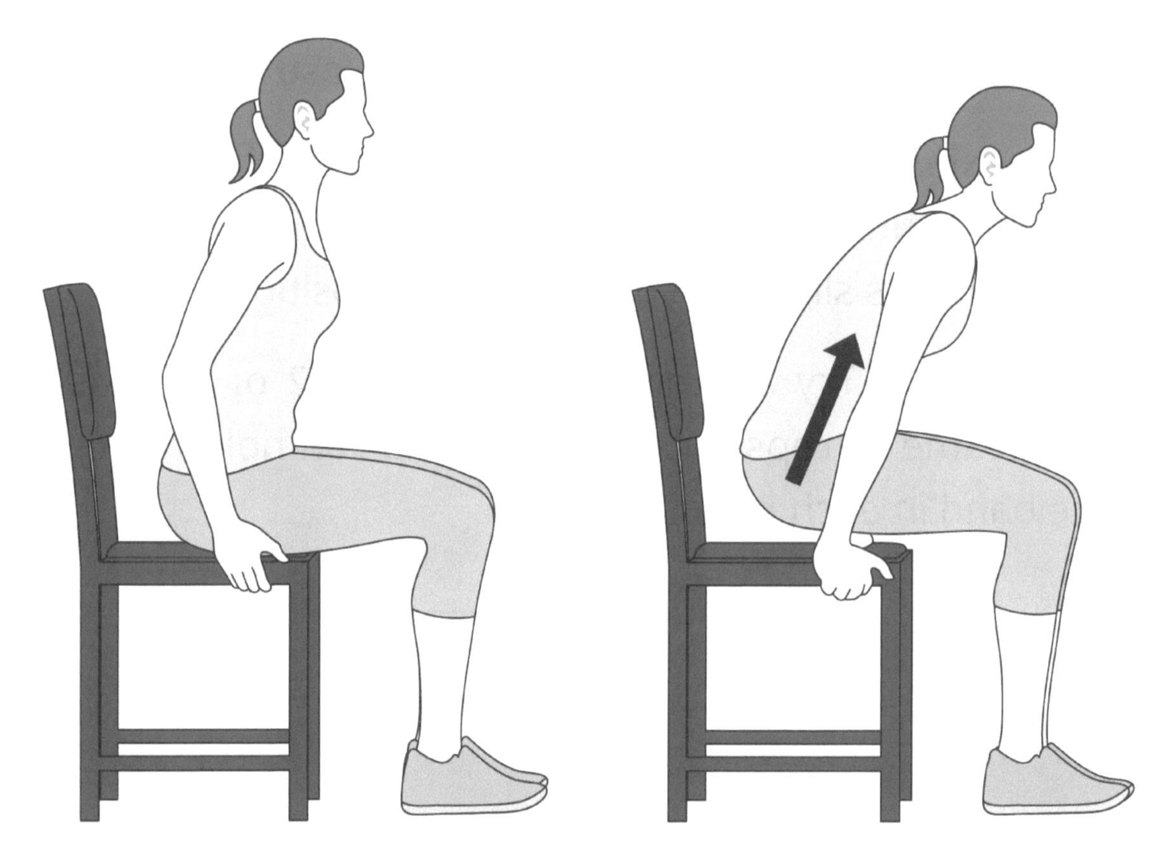

1. Begin by sitting upright in the middle of your chair with your shoulders down and back.

2. Place both feet underneath your knees, firmly planting them on the floor.

3. Rest your hands on the side of your chair beside your hips or on the armrest.

4. Bending at your hips, fold gently forward but keep your back straight.

5. Inhale and, as you breathe out, press down firmly through your hands, straightening your arms and lifting your buttocks off the chair.

6. Gently lower yourself down to sitting by bending your elbows.

7. Repeat for 8 reps.

Target: We want our elbows to be close to our bodies pushing with the heels of our palms.

Making it easier: You can support the lift by engaging your legs to assist or not fully lift off from sitting.

Adding difficulty: Using a chair with sturdy armrests allows you to raise higher, increasing the motion range. Only utilize your arm strength and increase the reps or add a tempo of 3232.

Bicep Curls

Our biceps are frequently engaged in daily activities, such as lifting objects, carrying groceries, or pushing or pulling open a door. Building strength in this muscle can help us perform these tasks with greater ease and less fatigue.

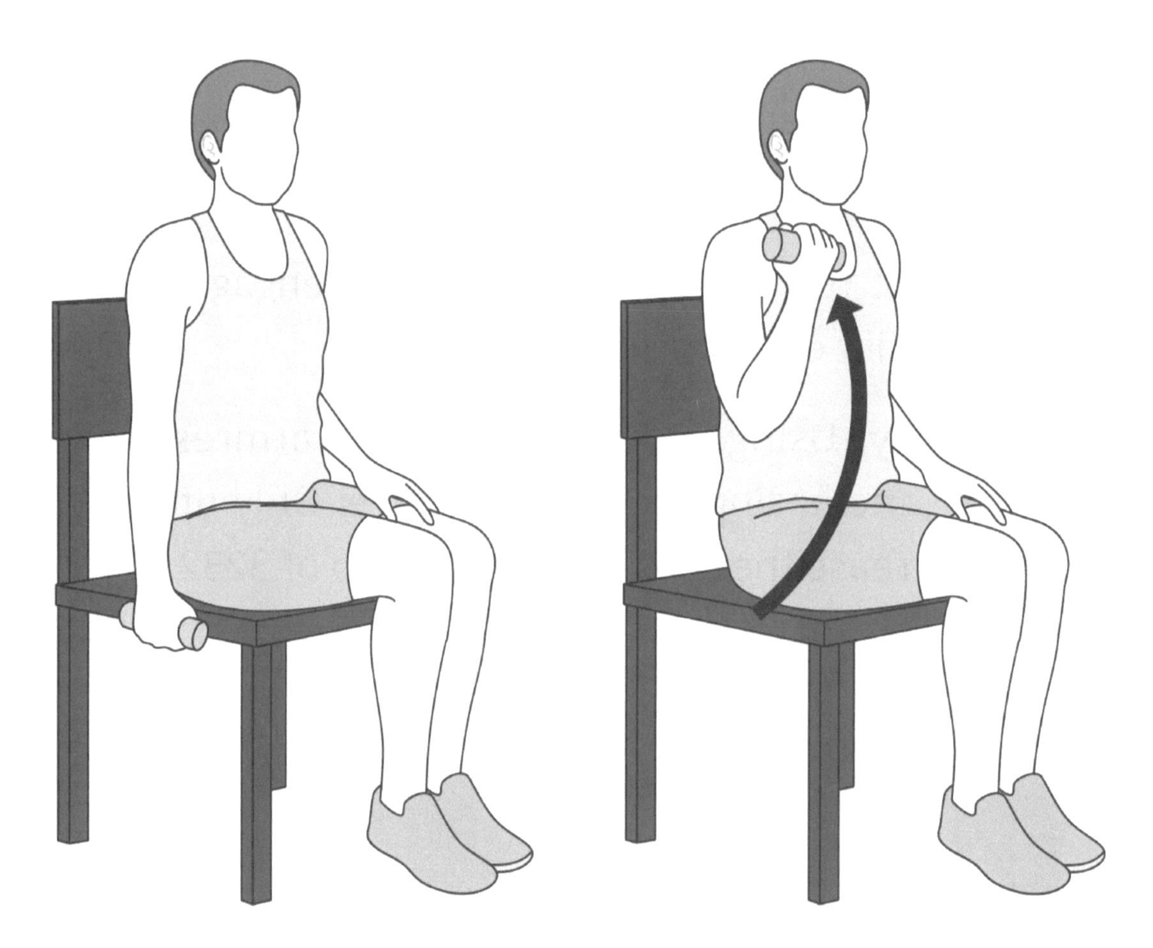

1. Begin by sitting upright in your chair with your shoulder blades down and back.

2. Your feet should be flat on the floor.

3. Inhale and bring your right arm to the side with your dumbbell in hand and your palm facing inward.

4. Inhale and rotate your wrist while you curl your arm from the elbow all the way to your shoulder.

5. Your dumbbells should touch your shoulders.

6. Exhale and lower your hand back down and uncurl them into their straight starting position.

7. Repeat for 8 reps.

8. Swap to your left side and perform 8 reps.

Target: We want to keep the upper arm and elbow stationary while smoothly bringing up and lowering our forearm with controlled movement.

Making it easier: Reduce the range of motion or reps and use lighter weights, resistance, or use without.

Adding difficulty: Try adding a tempo of 3232, increasing the weight or volume of reps. If using a resistance band, place the other end under your foot, ensuring it will not slip out. Another option is to perform the curl with a hammer grip with your palm facing inward.

Overhead Tricep Extension

This exercise strengthens the muscles in the shoulders and tricep arms muscles. This improves our ability for all grooming, dressing, grabbing objects from higher shelves, and activities that require pushing.

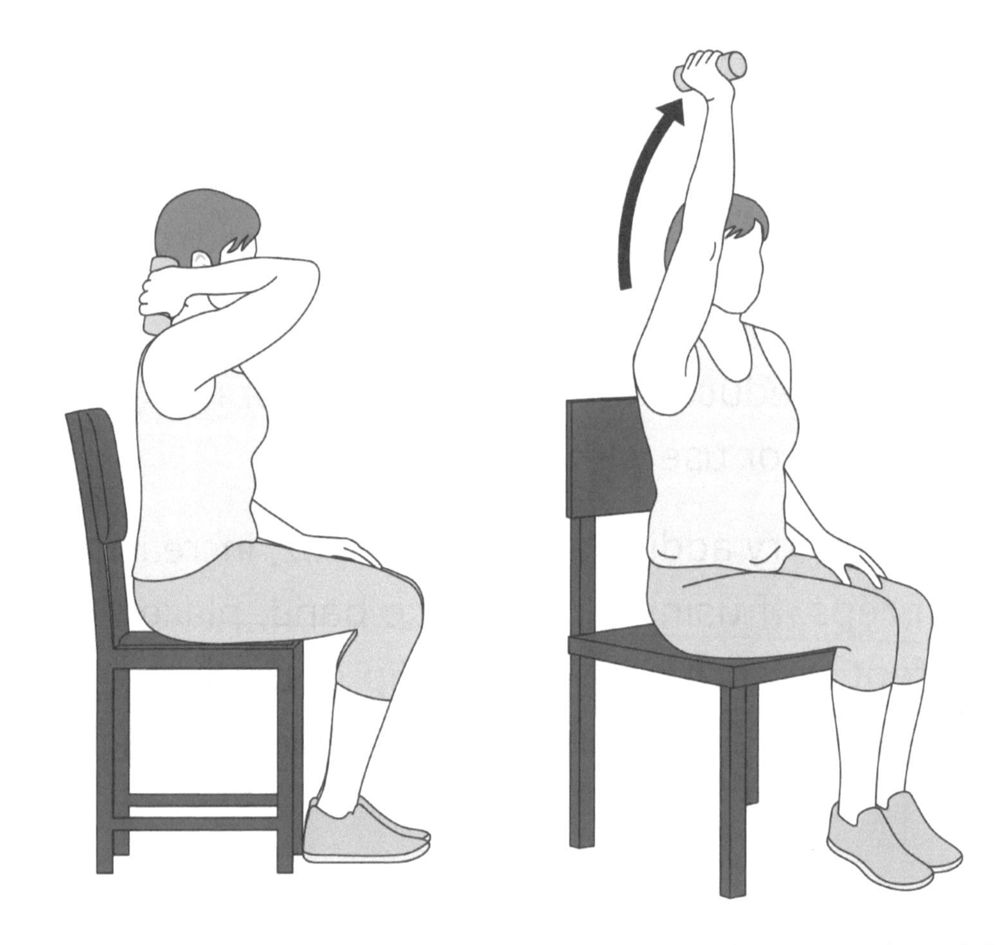

1. Begin by sitting upright in your chair with your shoulder blades down and back.

2. Your feet should be flat on the floor.

3. Grab a dumbbell in your right hand.

4. Bring your right hand with the dumbbell behind your right shoulder. Your upper arm and elbow should be in line with your ear.

5. Inhale and, as you exhale, straighten your elbow and arm above your head.

6. Inhale and gently lower your hand back down to your shoulder.

7. Repeat for 8 reps.

8. Repeat another 8 reps on your left side.

Target: We want to keep our back straight for the entire exercise with our elbows forward and close to our heads. Smooth and controlled motion up and down with manageable resistance gripping firmly to weight but not overly so.

Making it easier: Perform without weights, reduce the range of motion or volume of reps.

Adding difficulty: Alternative to the dumbbell weight, you can apply resistance using a resistance band by holding one end with your other hand resting at your hip on the side you are exercising. If you do not have any resistance equipment, you can also apply resistance with your other hand. Add a tempo of 3242, increasing the resistance or volume of reps.

Wrist Flexion and Extension

We may only sometimes consider how much we rely on our wrists for gardening, sports, music, pushing ourselves up from bed, chair, or even a fall. Our wrists also aid in our fine motor controls of opening doors, eating, cooking, using electronics, and knitting.

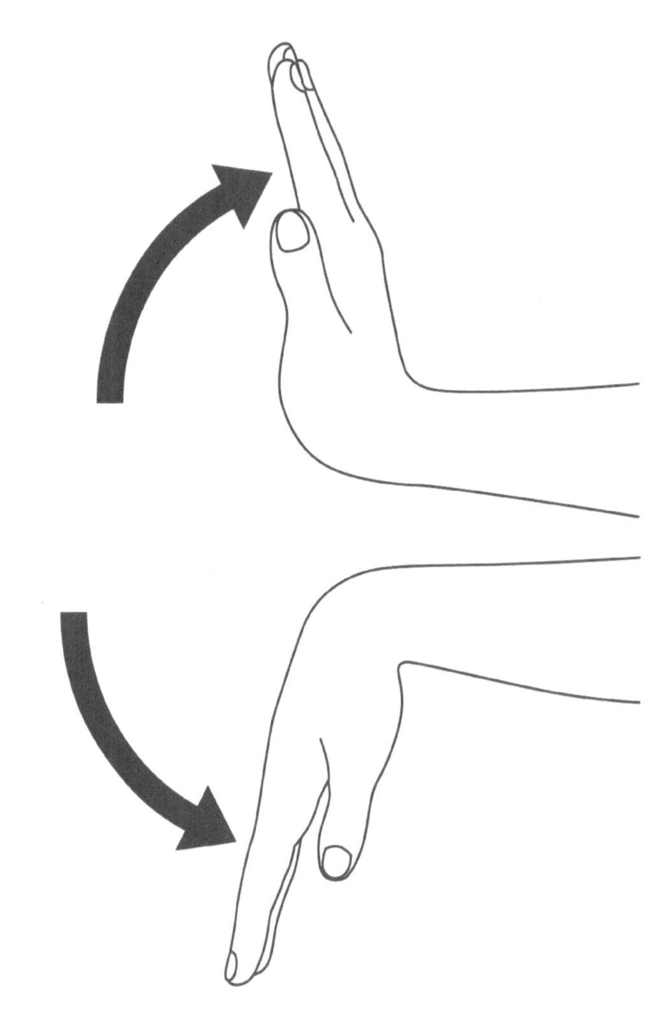

1. Begin by sitting upright in your chair at a table.
2. Place your arm on the table or thigh with your forearm on the surface with your palm facing downwards off the side of the tabletop or knee.
3. Bend at your wrist and move your fingers down toward the floor.

4. Bend at your wrist and move your fingers upward towards the ceiling.

5. Repeat for 8 repetitions.

6. Swap sides and repeat for 8 more reps.

Target: We want our wrist to move smoothly through its full range of motion while our forearm remains stationary and stable.

Making it easier: Reduce the volume of reps and your range of motion. You can also use your other hand to assist the movement.

Adding difficulty: Try the exercises while making a fist, holding weights, or applying resistance with your other hand. You can also add a tempo of 3333 or increase the volume of reps.

Squeeze

This exercise focuses on maintaining our grip strength and improving finger dexterity which is vital to our independence. It also has the added benefit of soothing Carpal Tunnel Syndrome and arthritis. It is also vital for gripping to support during a loss of balance.

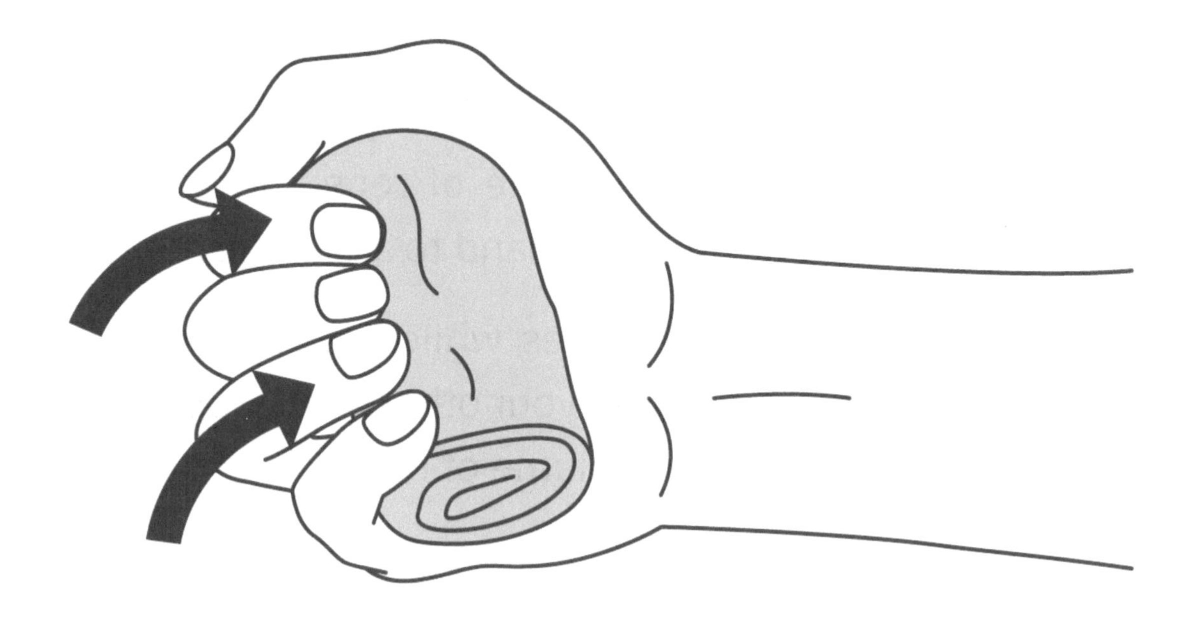

1. Begin by sitting upright in your chair with your shoulder blades down and back.
2. Your feet should be flat on the floor.
3. You will require an object to squeeze, such as a towel, tennis or stress ball, or hand exerciser.
4. Hold your item of choice with your hand in its neutral position.
5. Squeeze as hard as you can for three seconds.
6. Release your grip.

7. Repeat for 8 reps and swap sides.

Target: We want the object we are squeezing to feel comfortable in our hand, applying smooth and even pressure as we squeeze with our wrist in a straight position.

Making it easier: Reduce the volume of reps or time under tension. Depending on your object choice, you can heat or cool it to add a numbing or soothing sensation for sore arthritic joints.

Adding difficulty: Try alternating by squeezing with different fingers, such as pinky and ring, then ring and middle, then middle and index. You can also add a tempo of 3332 to increase the muscles' time under tension.

Now that we have our exercises for our extremities to our trunks, let us turn our attention to our main stabilizing muscles, our core.

Build Strength From Your Core

> It's easier to stay in shape if you never let yourself get out of shape in the first place.
>
> Bill Loguidice

Core strength is imperative for all our essential physical functions, from walking and balancing to standing and sitting. A strong core means a strong foundation for all our everyday movements.

The common misconception about our core is that it is only our abs. The core, however, is made up of a lot more different muscles, including the rectus abdominis (the front stomach muscles), the internal and external obliques (the muscles running along the sides), the transversus abdominis (the layer of muscle surrounding the spine), the hip muscles, and the lower back muscles (Weber, 2021).

When we reach our 30s, our core strength starts to decrease, resulting in the muscles around our spine and torso losing functionality, impacting our balance and mobility. It is the center point of our body and links our upper body to the lower body; therefore, we need to keep this link strong. I know we do not and cannot spend time thinking about how our bodies function and what each part does, but taking time to reflect on our physical elements can help us picture how and why our bodies work the way they do and how we can help them work correctly. We want to take notice before there is something wrong with our bodies. We want to preempt it.

Lifting, reaching, turning, and bending are all made easier by having a strong midline which means that all activities in daily life will still be manageable as we continue to age.

Core Strength and Balance Exercises

Safety moment: These exercises involve coordinated body movements designed to activate core muscles and may demand a certain level of balance. They are also generally used as moderate-intensity aerobic exercises and performed at a faster rhythm of motion. Always prioritize your comfort and safety:

- Ensure you stay within a range of motion that feels secure and avoids setting you off balance.
- Maintain proper form; if you're sacrificing technique, slow down.
- Pay attention to your body's signals. Adjust the tempo or take a break if your heartbeat feels irregular or your breathing becomes excessively labored.

Rowing Twists

This exercise promotes flexibility, strengthens the obliques, and enhances rotational mobility in the upper body. This motion helps to maintain a flexible spine and promotes better posture, which is crucial for daily activities and reducing back discomfort.

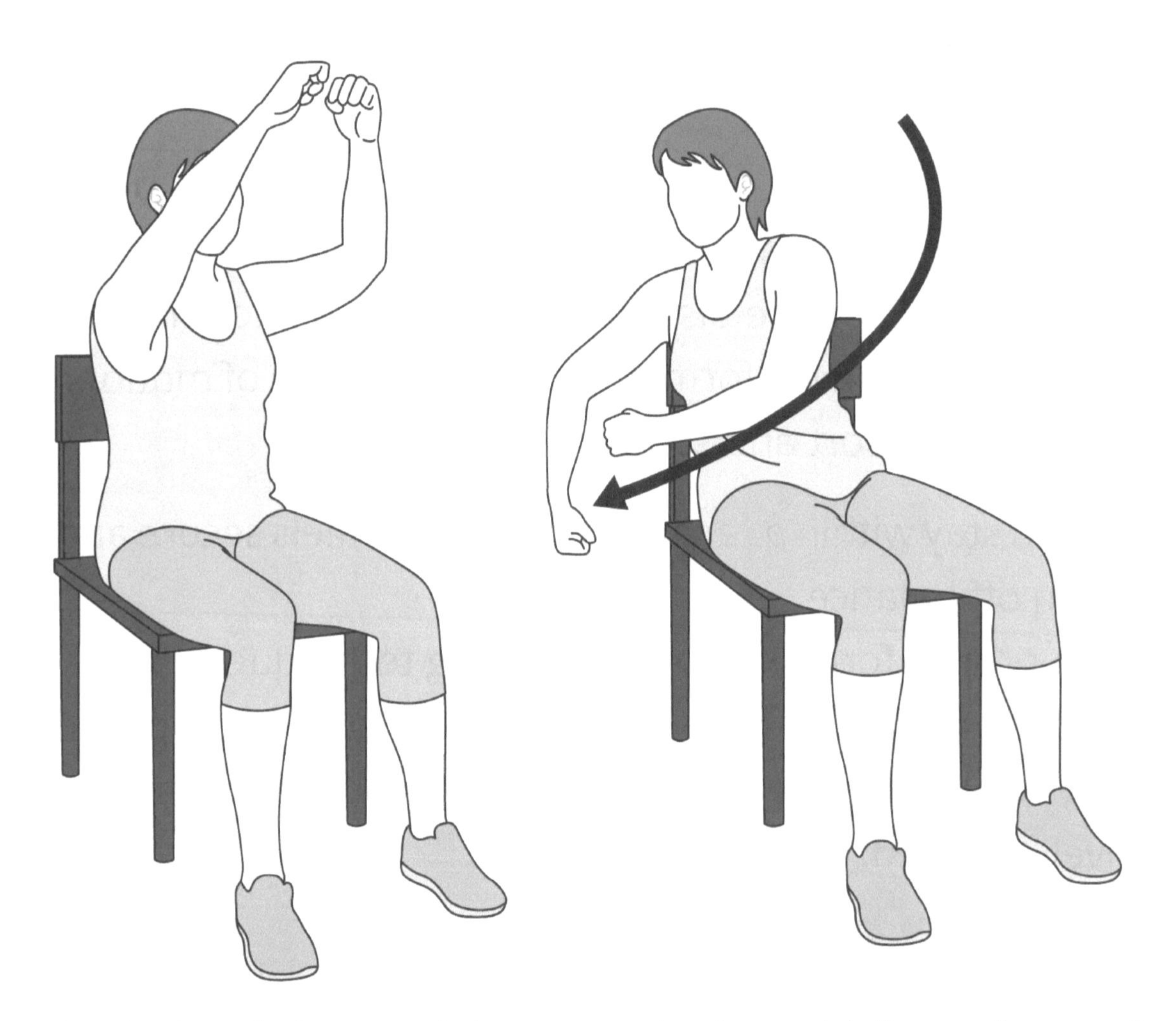

1. Begin by sitting upright towards the middle or front of your chair with your shoulders down and back.
2. Place both feet underneath your knees, firmly planting them on the floor.
3. Lean back but do not let your back touch the back of the chair if you can.

4. Inhale as you raise your hands in front of your face like you are holding a paddle with the right hand over the other.

5. Exhale and twist to your left, rotating your shoulders and bringing your hands down to your left side.

6. Inhale as you raise your hands in front of your face like you are holding a paddle with the left hand over the other.

7. Exhale and twist to your right, rotating your shoulders and bringing your hands down to your right side.

8. Repeat for rowing alternately left and right for 8 reps.

Target: We want to imagine ourselves paddling a boat across the water, rotating from the core as we push our oar down and back.

Making it easier: You can lean against the chair, limit how far you take the movement, or hold the chair with the hand for the side you are rotating toward for stability.

Adding difficulty: Try adding weights in both hands orientated so they touch end to end, or hold a taught resistance band or towel as an oar for the movements. Additionally, you can either speed up the rows to increase aerobic intensity or slow it down by adding a tempo of 3232.

Seated Jumping Jacks

This exercise offers cardiovascular benefits similar to standing jumping jacks without the jolting impact on the lower joints. It also aids in enhancing arm and leg coordination, promoting circulation, and building endurance.

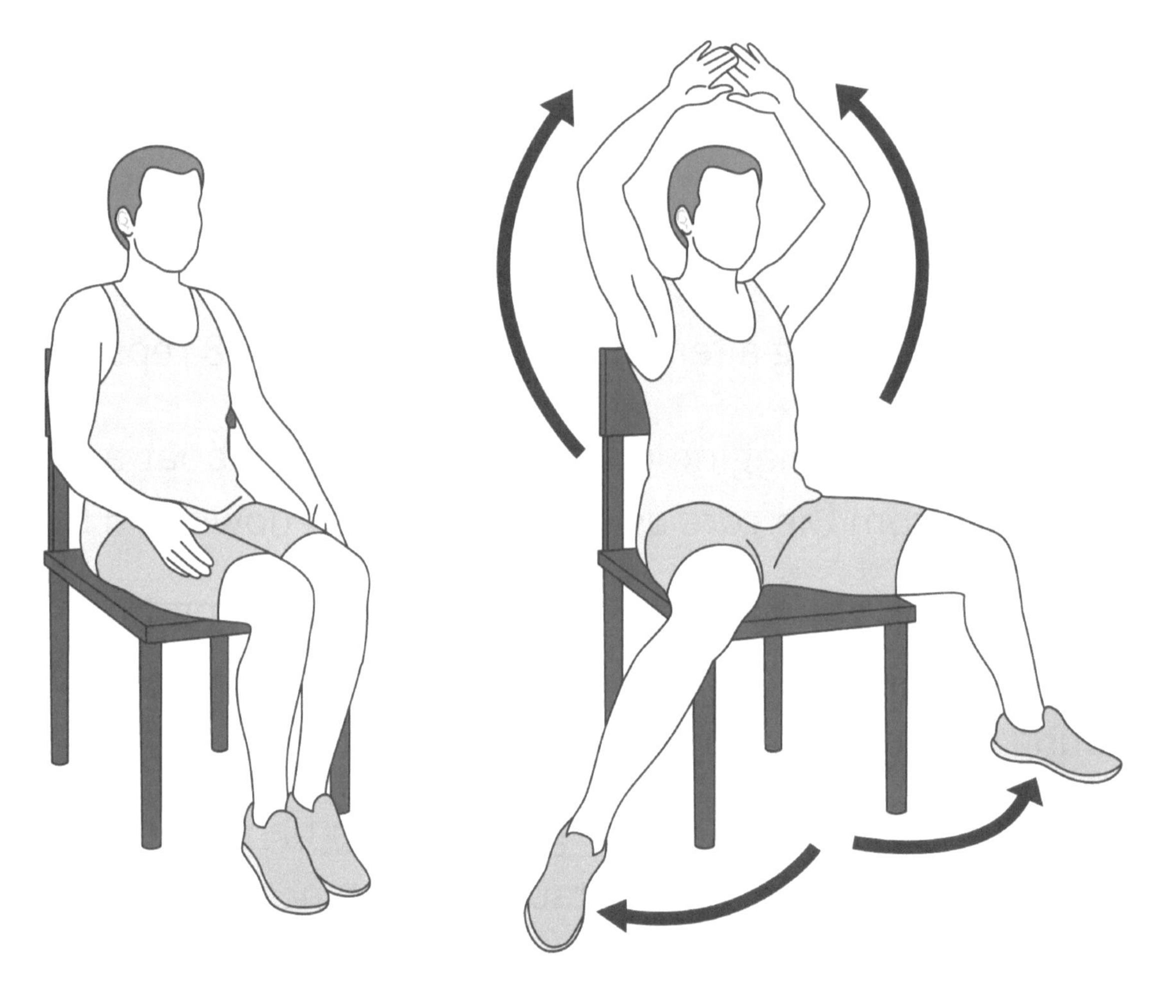

1. Begin by sitting upright towards the front of your chair with your shoulders down and back. Ensure your chair is stable and not in danger of tipping forward with your weight.

2. Keep your arms to your side and your feet together in front of your chair.

3. Inhale and swing your arms upwards and overhead as you si-

multaneously step both legs outwards to shoulder width apart.

4. Return to your starting position by bringing your hands back down to your sides and feet together.

5. Repeat for 10 reps.

Target: We want to focus on synchronizing your arm and leg movements, creating a fluid motion as we expand and return.

Making it easier: To add more stability, only raise and extend your arm and leg on one side at a time, holding the chair with the other hand and firmly planting your other foot on the ground. You can also limit the range of motion or reduce the volume of reps.

Adding difficulty: Increase the tempo to step up your heart rate or slow down the tempo to 2121, pausing at the open and close of the movement.

Bicycle

This exercise engages the quadriceps, hamstrings, hip flexors, rectus abdominis, and obliques. This movement replicates the pedaling motion, promoting better leg coordination and hip flexibility while improving leg mobility and promoting blood circulation.

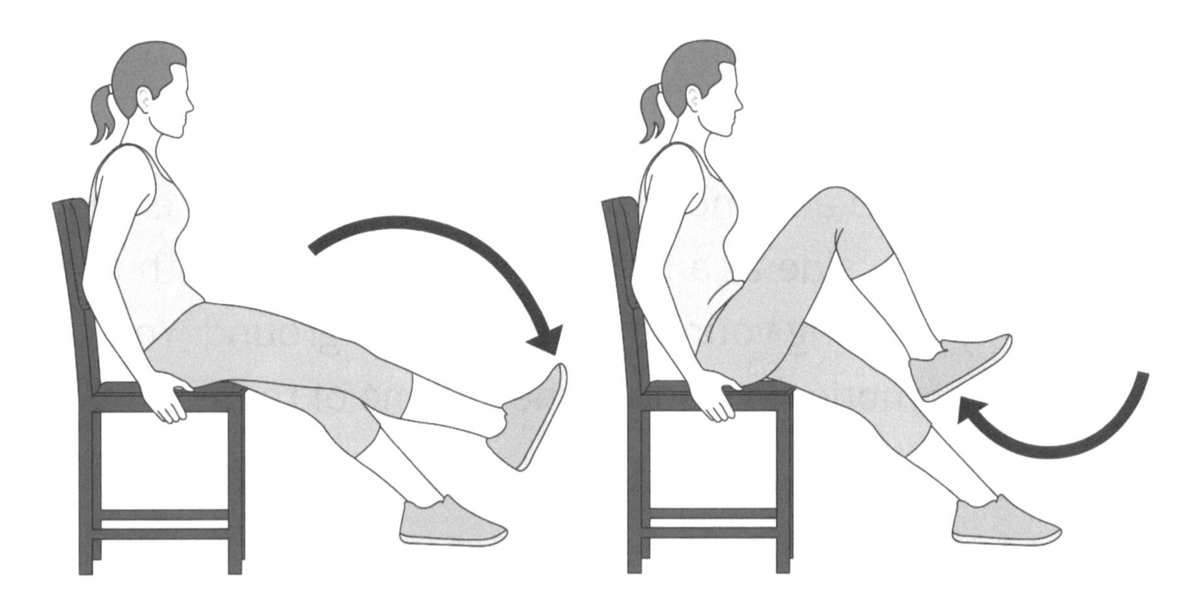

1. Begin by sitting upright and slightly forward in your chair with your shoulders down and back. Ensure your chair is stable and not in danger of tipping forward with your weight.

2. Hold on to the sides of your chair and lean back into the chair's backrest with your feet stretched out in front of you.

3. Keep breathing throughout this entire exercise.

4. Raise your left leg and make a large circle with your foot, bringing it down and toward you, then up and arc your foot forward until your leg is outstretched again.

5. Repeat this cycle for 6 rotations.

6. Now reverse the rotation, make a large circle with your foot, arcing it up and toward you, then down and forward, kicking your foot forward until your leg is outstretched again.

7. Repeat this cycle for 6 rotations.

8. Repeat the entire series on the right leg, 6 rotations down and back, then 6 rotations up and back.

Target: We want to concentrate on the circular motion of the leg, aiming for smooth and consistent circular rotations. Think that you are pedaling a recumbent bicycle.

Making it easier: Limit the range of motion by making smaller circles with your legs or bring your resting leg closer for added stability.

Adding difficulty: Try leaning forward when your knee is close to your body to crunch and engage the core more. You can also attempt to cycle both legs simultaneously for added coordination and core engagement.

Hip Flexor Exercise

This exercise aids in opening up the hip joints, countering the effects of prolonged sitting. Strengthening the hip flexors can also improve stability during walking.

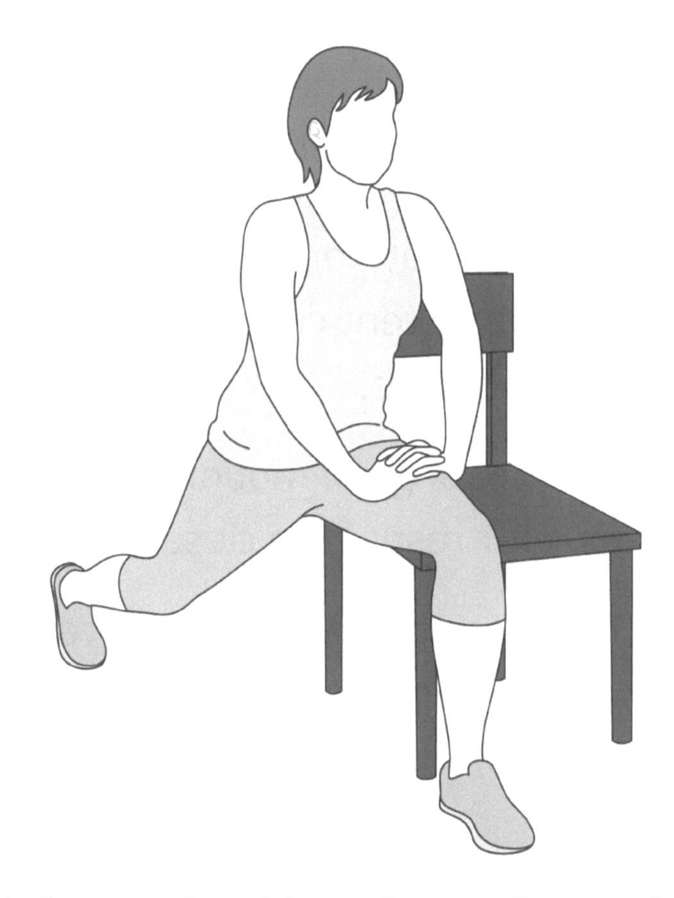

1. Begin by sitting on the side or front of your chair with one thigh off and one thigh on the chair.

2. The leg still on the chair will be in front of the chair at a 90° angle with your foot flat on the ground.

3. Bring your other foot as far back behind you as you can. You should feel a stretch in the front of your outstretched leg.

4. Breathe deeply and hold that position for 20 seconds.

5. Repeat on the other side.

Target: We want to focus on a gentle stretch in the hip area and outstretched leg, keeping the spine straight and chest open.

Making it easier: Limit how far back you extend your leg and lean closer to the center of the chair for more stability holding the chair's backrest for support.

Adding difficulty: Increase the time you hold the stretch. You can also lift the outstretched foot up and down for several reps to engage the surrounding muscles around the hip flexor.

Flutter Kicks

Flutter kicks primarily target the lower abdominal muscles while promoting leg coordination and circulation. This is instrumental in enhancing core stability and strength necessary for day-to-day movements.

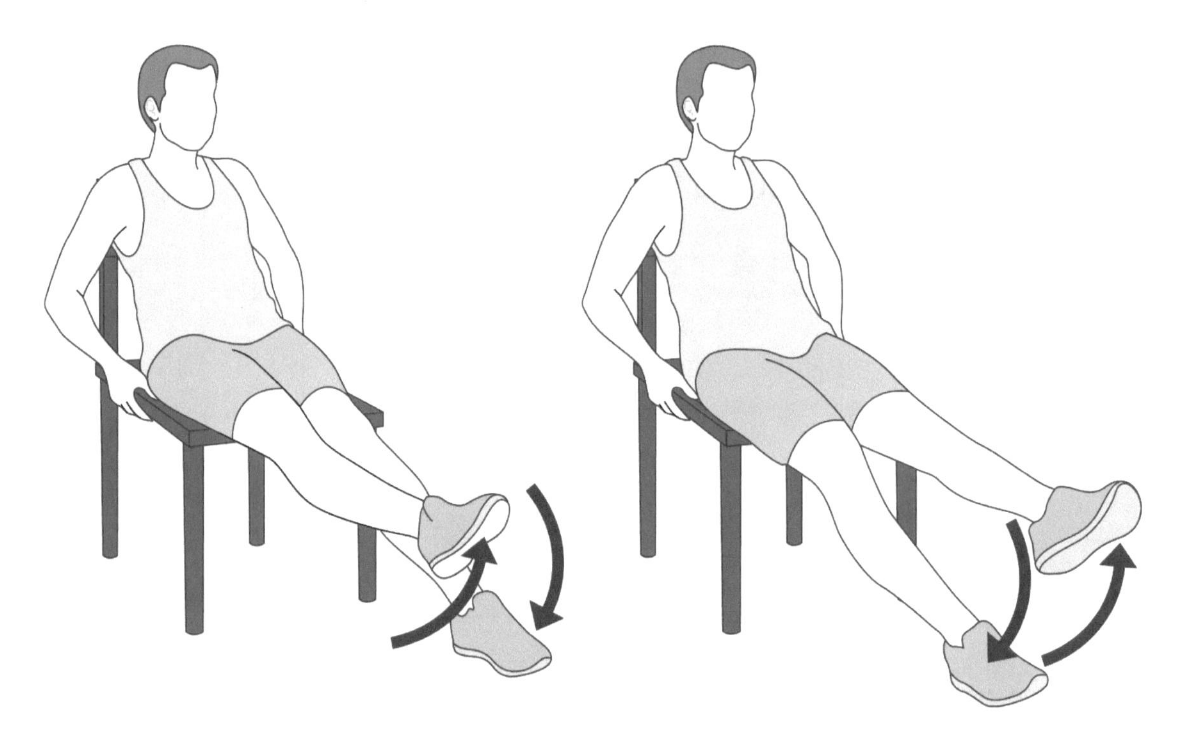

1. Begin by sitting upright and slightly forward in your chair with your shoulders down and back. Ensure your chair is stable and not in danger of tipping forward with your weight.

2. Hold on to the sides of your chair and lean back with your feet stretched out in front of you.

3. Keep breathing throughout the movement.

4. Raise your feet while keeping your legs straight and preventing them from touching the ground. Alternate raising and lowering your left and right foot in small movements.

5. Continue for 30 seconds.

Target: We want to keep a rhythmic and steady motion, alternate elevating our legs without allowing them to touch the ground. The emphasis should be on maintaining a tight core, ensuring our back is supported, and our movements are precise and controlled.

Making it easier: Bend your knees slightly, decreasing the lever length and making lifting and lowering the legs easier. Reduce the elevation of the kicks so you're moving your feet just a couple of inches up and down.

Adding difficulty: Incorporate different rhythms, such as performing a set of quick, shallow kicks followed by slower, more deliberate, and higher kicks.

Seated Half Rollbacks

This exercise emphasizes spinal flexibility and core engagement. Such movements help counteract the forward hunch often developed over the years and improve overall posture.

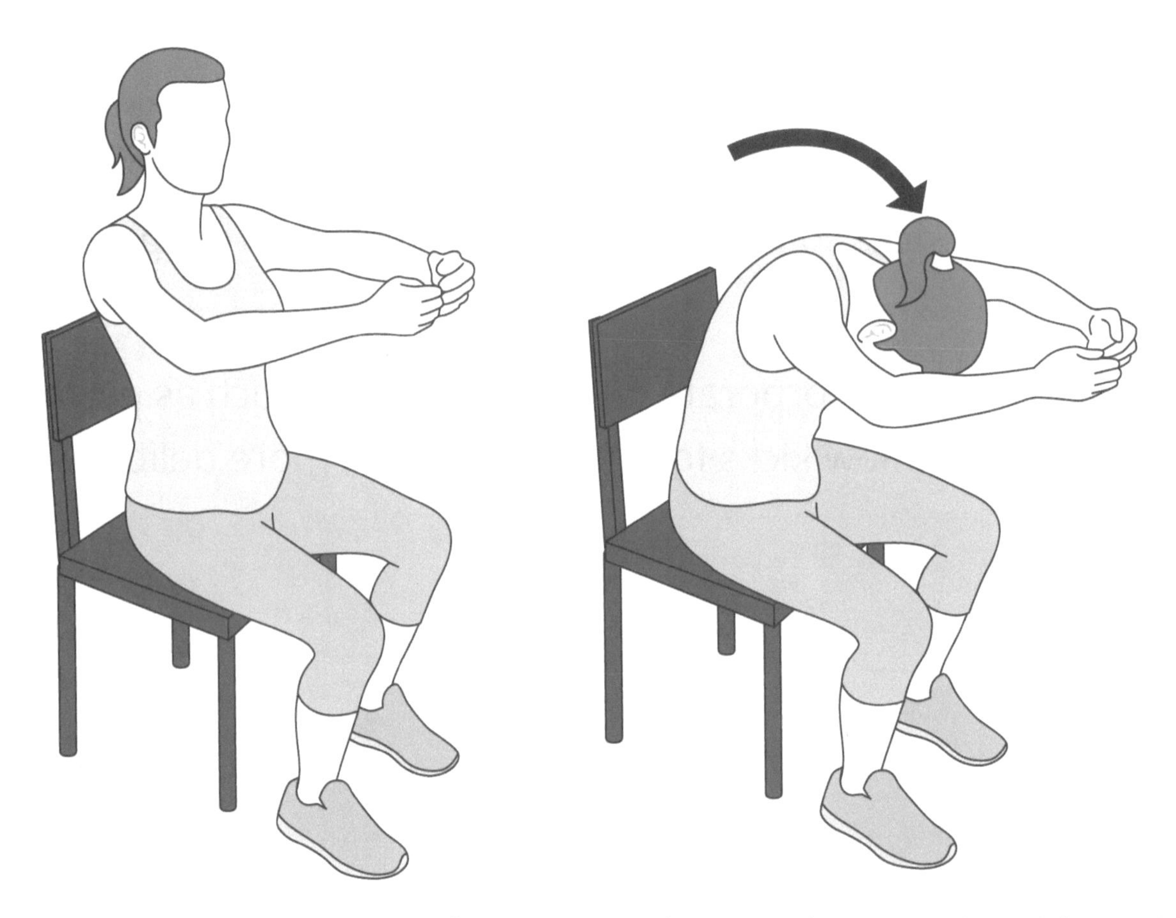

1. Begin by sitting upright in your chair with your shoulders down and back.

2. Place your legs in front of you with your knees bent at 90°. Your feet should be flat on the floor.

3. Raise your hands in front of you and grasp your hands together, creating a circle with your arms.

4. Ensure that your back is straight.

5. Inhale and, as you exhale, roll your chin towards your chest. Think of scooping up your abs.

6. Go as far as you feel comfortable, engage your midline, and slowly move back toward your upright position.

7. Repeat for 8 reps.

Target: We want to focus on engaging our core as we curl our backs forward and scoop our core in and up, pulling our belly button back towards our spine.

Making it easier: Unclasp your hands, rest them on your thighs for added support and guidance, and limit how far your spine curves.

Adding difficulty: Slow the movement down by adding a tempo of 4444 or lift the arms as you move back, keeping them in line with your head. This changes your center of gravity and requires more core strength to stabilize.

Leg Taps

Leg taps enhance lower body coordination while activating the quadriceps and hip flexors. Improved quad strength aids in activities like standing up from a seated position or climbing stairs.

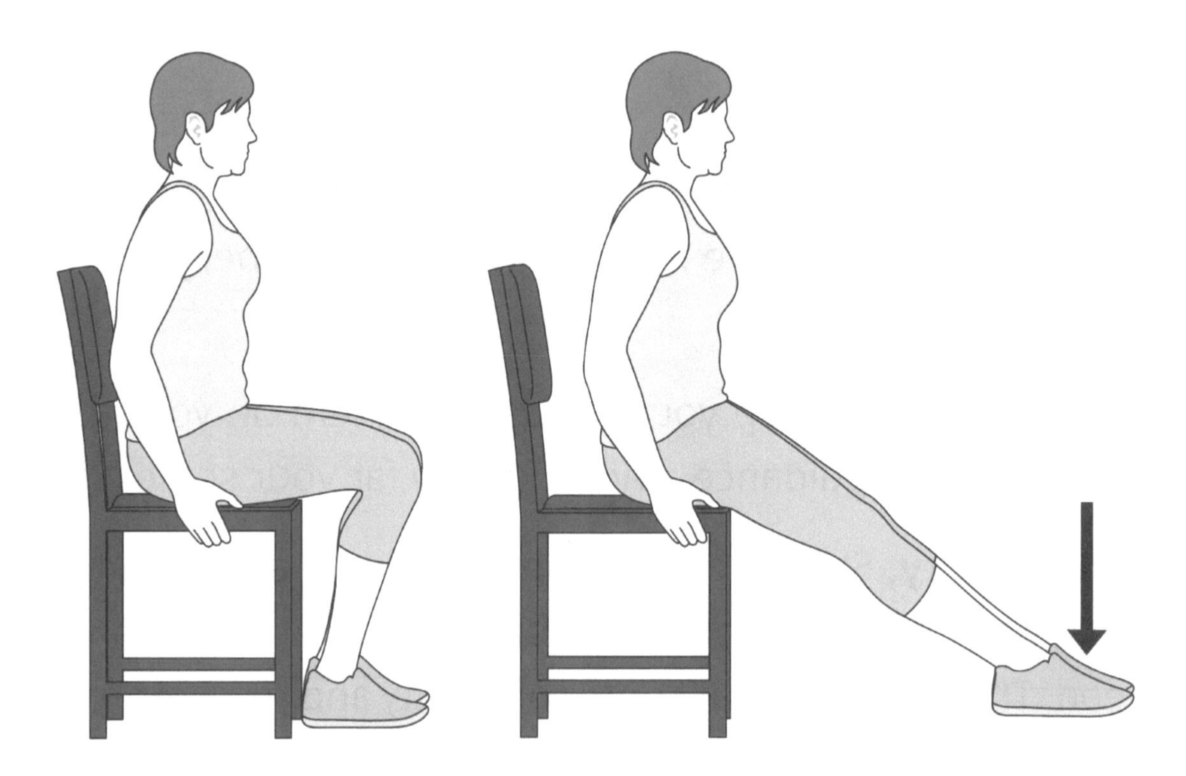

1. Begin by sitting upright in your chair with your shoulders down and back.
2. Place your feet flat on the ground in front of your chair at a 90° angle.
3. Hold onto the sides of your chair for support.
4. Exhale, lift and extend both legs out in front of you and lightly tap them to the floor.
5. Inhale, lift and bring your feet back and tap the starting point.
6. Repeat for 8 reps.

Target: We want to focus on controlled leg movements, hovering our feet off the ground as we sweep them forward and back, gently tapping them to the floor while maintaining a consistent rhythm and ensuring our core remains engaged throughout the motion.

Making it easier: For stability, only extend one leg at a time utilizing the other leg for balance. Also, reduce how far you stretch your legs outward.

Adding difficulty: Try slowing the movement down by adding a tempo of 3131 or adding a double tap on the floor after extending the legs before pulling them back.

Now that we have pushed through all of the core exercises, let us take a moment to slow down our heart rates, wind down our tired muscles and take some much-needed breaths in the next chapter, Cooldown and Recovery.

Cooldown & Recovery

> Once you are exercising regularly, the hardest thing is to stop it.
>
> Erin Gray

Like a good warm-up routine, a good cooldown routine is just as important as the workout. There are several benefits to cooling down.

Your cooldown will help lower your heart rate and return your body to its pre-exercise state. You want to encourage your heart rate, breathing, and temperature to return to normal.

Generally, it would be best to focus your cooldown stretches and movements on the muscle group you worked on in your session. And remember, it does not have to be long—a quick 10-minute cooldown is more than sufficient.

Cooldown Routines

Cooldown Routine One

1. Begin by sitting upright in your chair with your shoulders down and back.

2. Let your arms hang to the side of your body.

3. Inhale and shrug your shoulders, raising your arms as you rotate them backward in a circular motion.

4. Keep your arms straight and close to your body as you do so. Repeat these backward rotations for 20 repetitions.

5. Return to a neutral position and repeat forward for 20 repetitions.

6. Bring your arms up to the side of your body so that they are in line with your shoulders and your palms are facing the ceiling.

7. Inhale and bring your palms together up overhead.

8. Bend both elbows so that your arms touch the back of your neck. Hold this position for five breaths.

9. Release and repeat this movement another two times for three repetitions.

10. Return to your neutral seated position. Place your right hand on your left hip, and your left hand will be behind you.

11. As you breathe out, gently twist your torso and look over your left hip. Hold for three breaths and return to neutral.

12. Place your left hand on your right hip, and your right hand will be behind you.

13. As you exhale, gently twist your torso and look over your right hip. Hold for three breaths and return to neutral.

14. Repeat twice more on each side for a total of three repetitions.
15. Move to the front of your chair, ensuring you are stable and balanced.
16. Inhale and, on your exhale, extend your left leg out in front of you while keeping your right leg bent at a 90° angle.
17. Place your hands on the thigh of your right leg and slowly relax into the stretch by allowing your chest and torso to drop downwards gently. Hold for three to five breaths and release. As you exhale, sink deeper into the stretch.
18. Return to your neutral seated position and repeat on the other side.
19. Alternate and repeat this two more times for a total of three repetitions.
20. Place both feet firmly on the floor with your ankles under your knees at a 90° angle.
21. Place your left ankle on your right knee. You can straighten out your right leg or keep it bent if necessary.
22. Inhale and, as you bend from your hips, exhale and gently bend forward, bringing your chest to your leg.
23. Hold for five breaths and repeat on the other side. As you breathe in and out, sink deeper into the stretch.

Cooldown Routine Two

1. Begin by sitting upright in your chair with your shoulders down and back.
2. Interlace your fingers and bring your palms upwards to face the ceiling.
3. Exhale and press your hands upward and backward as far as you feel comfortable. Keep your spine straight.
4. Hold for five breaths and return to neutral.
5. Shift yourself toward the front of your chair, keeping your shoulders down and back.
6. Keep your feet flat on the floor with your ankles under your knees.
7. Inhale and raise your left leg, bringing your left thigh up towards your chest. Keep your back straight.
8. You can use your arms to gently pull it closer to your torso until you reach a comfortable position. Exhale as you do so.
9. Hold for three breaths and release.
10. Repeat on the other side. Alternate for six alternating repetitions.
11. Get off your chair and stand behind it using the backrest as support.

12. Bend your right leg and bring your heel to your buttocks using a hand to help hold it up. Hold this position for 30 seconds.

13. Lower your leg and repeat on the other side.

Cooldown Routine Three

1. Begin by sitting upright towards the front of your chair with your shoulders down and back.
2. Your feet should be underneath your knees and your arms at your side.
3. Lift your left leg, keeping your knee bent, and raise your right leg. You are replicating a marching movement. Lower your leg and arm and repeat on the other side.
4. March for 30 seconds.
5. Return to your neutral position with both feet flat on the ground.
6. Inhale and bring your right ankle up onto your left knee. Rest your hands on your shins.
7. Remain sitting up tall and, as you exhale, gently fold forward from your hips, drawing your chest to your shin.
8. You can increase the stretch by gently pushing down on your right knee.
9. Hold for 30 seconds.
10. Repeat on the other side.
11. Return to neutral and spread your legs outwards, keeping your knees bent and in line with your toes.

12. Put your hands on your knees and push them outward. You should feel a stretch in your inner thighs.

13. Hold for 30 seconds, ensuring that you are not leaning forward but are maintaining a straight and upright back.

14. Return to your neutral position with your feet flat on the floor and your knees over your ankles.

15. Extend your left leg in front of you and raise your heel off the floor. Flex your foot to point your toes forward, and slowly rotate your ankle clockwise.

16. Repeat for 20 rotations.

17. Repeat in the anticlockwise direction.

18. Return your feet to neutral and repeat on the other side.

Breathing Exercises

In addition to the cooldown routines, I recommend Breathing exercises to help calm the heart and promote the resaturation of oxygen to the muscles. As we age, we tend to switch from taking deep breaths that fully engage our diaphragm to shallow breaths that only engage our upper chest. Taking 5-10 minutes to sit and focus on breathing can be phenomenal for our recovery and overall wellness. Focusing on breathing also helps calm your mind and helps you feel relaxed. If you feel lightheaded or dizzy at any point while performing a breathing exercise, revert to your regular breathing pattern.

Diaphragm Breathing

Otherwise known as belly breathing or abdominal breathing is a type of breathing that engages the diaphragm to fully expand the lungs allowing for better oxygen transfer and removal of waste gasses. This breathing exercise aims to keep your chest stationary while your belly extends and retracts with your breathing.

1. Sit in your chair with your knees bent and your shoulders, neck, and head relaxed.

2. Place one hand at the center of your upper chest and place your other hand on your belly, just below your rib cage.

3. Breathe slowly in through your nose, focusing on pushing your stomach out against your lower hand. Your upper hand should remain motionless.

4. Tighten your stomach muscles so that your stomach moves

back toward your spine as you exhale through pursed lips. The hand on your upper chest should remain motionless.

5. Repeat for 5-10 minutes.

With enough practice, you will not need to use your hands as guides to help you visualize and direct your core as you breathe. Ideally, we should always be breathing through our diaphragms; with enough concentrated breathing exercises, it will come more naturally to you.

Box Breathing

No, I do not mean breathing while stuck in a box. Box Breathing refers to the symmetrical breathing pattern at a 4444 tempo as follows.

1. Breathe in slowly through your nose for 4 seconds.

2. Hold your breath for 4 seconds.

3. Breathe out slowly through pursed lips for 4 seconds.

4. Hold your breath for 4 seconds.

5. Repeat for 5-10 minutes.

Box breathing is excellent for slowing the heart rate and stabilizing blood pressure. By focusing on the steady count, your mind clears away distractions and improves your concentration. As your heart rate stabilizes, you can switch from a mental count to keeping time with your heartbeats.

4-7-8 Breathing

Another alternative to box breathing is breathing at a 478 tempo. Dr. Andrew Weil has popularized the 478 tempo breathing. Sit with your back flat against your chair's backrest. Place the tip of your tongue against the ridge of tissue just behind your upper front teeth, and keep it there throughout the entire exercise. You will be exhaling through your mouth around your tongue; try pursing your lips slightly if this seems awkward.

1. Exhale completely through your mouth, making a whoosh sound.

2. Close your mouth and inhale quietly through your nose to a mental count of four.

3. Hold your breath for a count of seven.

4. Exhale completely through your mouth, making a whoosh sound to a count of eight. This is one breath.

5. Now inhale again and repeat the cycle three more times for a total of four breaths.

If you have trouble holding your breath, speed the exercise up but keep to the ratio of 4:7:8 for the three phases. With practice, you can slow it down and get used to inhaling and exhaling more deeply. (Weil, A. n.d)

Post-workout Recovery

Hydration

We talked about staying hydrated before, during, and after workout sessions. I want to reiterate and stress how important making sure you drink fluids after your workout. You may not always be able to tell how much water you lost during your workout. For me, I am afraid to say, I sweat buckets. Even though we drink before and during our workout, we need to drink even more after to help aid in recovery. Water supports every metabolic function in your body essential for recovery. Ensuring you stay hydrated also help prevents muscle cramps, fatigue, and low blood pressure post-workout.

Nutrition

Refueling the body with protein, carbohydrates, fats, dairy, and colorful fruits is an excellent way to aid your post-workout recovery. Proper nutrition is crucial to workout recovery, which remains valid as we age. Our bodies burn through essential nutrients that our diets need to replenish. Here are some nutrient-rich foods and beverages that can be beneficial post-workout:

1. **Protein**: Protein is the main ingredient in muscle recovery and growth. It helps repair the muscle tissues that get broken down when we exercise. Choose lean protein sources like chicken, turkey, fish, and eggs or plant-based proteins like lentils, chickpeas, or tofu. They even have protein powders or shakes for a quick, easy post-workout meal or snack.

1. **Carbohydrates**: Carbs help replenish the glycogen used as energy during your workout. Whole grain bread, brown rice, quinoa, oatmeal, and fruits like bananas, berries, or apples are all excellent sources of healthy carbs.

2. **Healthy Fats**: Monounsaturated and polyunsaturated fats are good for heart health and can help control inflammation. Avocados, nuts, seeds, and oily fish such as salmon are all high in these healthy fats.

3. **Dairy and Dairy Alternatives**: Milk and yogurt are good protein and carbohydrate sources, making them excellent post-workout snacks. They are also a source of calcium, which is vital for bone health.

4. **Colorful Fruits and Vegetables**: These are high in antioxidants and can help reduce inflammation. They are also a good source of vitamins and minerals that aid recovery and overall health.

An option for a post-workout meal could be grilled chicken with quinoa and steamed vegetables or a protein smoothie with a scoop of protein powder, a banana, a handful of spinach, and some almond milk.

Remember, nutritional needs can vary widely based on factors like the intensity and duration of the workout, underlying health conditions, and personal preferences. It's always a good idea to consult with a registered dietitian.

The last thing we need to do is construct our plan by putting together all the exercises to increase and maintain our physical strength as we progress week by week.

The next chapter will take you through this process. This is one of my most exciting steps when putting together a workout plan, and I love the process of building an exercise program. I hope you have as much fun as I do.

Building Your 7-Day Routine

I understand you may feel overwhelmed or apprehensive about putting an exercise plan together; that is natural. I am confident that we can tackle this task together.

Which muscles to work when? How many days a week to train? When should we do strength versus balance training?

Try not to overthink things. We will streamline the process and have you set up to reach your goals by breaking things down day by day.

Exercise Guidelines

According to the CDC (2019), adults who are 65 years old or older should aim for 150 minutes of exercise a week.

Moderate-Intensity Aerobic Exercise

The routines here strive for at least 150 minutes of moderate-intensity aerobic exercise spread across the week. Such consistency is beneficial for cardiovascular health and promotes increased stamina. Engaging in these routines will ensure that your heart rate gets the gentle elevation it needs and that you remain in the optimal intensity zone, striking a challenging yet manageable rhythm.

You can gauge whether you are at a moderate-intensity level by paying attention to your breathing and heart rate. You will find that these will elevate slightly, and you will begin to sweat. If you wanted to talk, you could still hold a conversation.

Looking at it from a sliding scale of 1–10, where 1 is sitting, and 10 is a full-out effort, a moderate-intensity pace would sit between 5–6.

Strength or Resistance Training

Using your own body weight, or incorporating weights and resistance bands into your training routine, is crucial for maintaining muscle mass and bone density.

You want to ensure that you work out all the major muscle groups, such as your legs, hips, back, chest, abdomen, shoulders, and arms. Aim to do 2–3 sets of muscle-building activity with 8–12 repetitions per set, two days a week (CDC, 2019).

Balance and Flexibility Exercises

Balance exercises will help you maintain a fulfilling and functional lifestyle by ensuring that your day-to-day activities remain achievable. Balance and flexibility training also reduces the risk of falls, fractures, and other injuries.

The U.S. Department of Health and Human Services (n.d.) recommends that you do three sessions a week of balance activities.

While working on your balance, you should also be aware of your flexibility, which may decrease with age. We always want to ensure we can move our joints and limbs through their full range of motion.

Progress at Your Own Pace

Fitness is a journey, not a destination. While the CDC's and the U.S. Department of Health and Human Services guidelines set a standard for health and fitness, it's important to remember that everyone's path to achieving these targets will be unique.

Starting small can be a game-changer. If you're new to exercising or getting back into it after a break, it's perfectly okay, to begin with just one or two exercises a couple of times a week. It will help your body adjust, reduce the risk of injuries, and prevent feelings of overwhelm or burnout. Over time, as your endurance and energy levels grow, you can gradually increase the intensity and frequency of your workouts.

The goal is consistent progression. Eventually, you will gain the stamina to engage in an entire workout or even exercise daily. But even on days when you feel you're not up to a full session, remember that something is always better than nothing. A few stretches can still contribute to your overall well-being.

Listen to your body. There will be days when you feel invincible and other days when rest might be the best choice. No matter how small, every step you take is towards a healthier you. Adapt the exercises to where you are now and allow yourself to grow.

Your Workout Plans

Each session will begin with either a general whole-body or targeted warm-up concentrating on a particular muscle group. Again, you can choose which one you want for the day—be creative, as the warm-up primes your body to work out but also infuses variety into your program.

This book is structured so that you have a choice of seven exercises from each body chapter. All you have to do is select one exercise from each body section chapter, and you will have a workout that works your whole body.

Alternatively, you could split your workouts, focusing on specific muscle groups. For instance, you could focus on the ankles and legs on Monday, while Tuesday, are neck and shoulders.

While there are many ways to tailor a routine, I recommend incorporating an exercise from each body section. This approach keeps your workouts diverse and ensures no single muscle group becomes overworked or leaves you fatigued. You also get balance training, strength training, and aerobic exercise throughout the week, meeting the agency's guidelines.

Your sessions will end with one of the cooldown routines. Feel free to add or omit any sections to your plan but ensure you complete a cooldown before ending your session. It is good for your recovery and will return your mind and body to a pre-exercise mode.

Stretches are integrated into every warm-up and cooldown, but you can add dynamic stretches from any body section chapters to your warm-up, cooldown, or throughout the day whenever you need them.

Seven-Day Whole Body Workout Program

This example takes one exercise from each body chapter for five exercises with a warm-up and cooldown of your choice. It cycles through all the exercises throughout the week, balancing all muscle groups and training. You can use this one or mix and match to suit your needs.

Monday

1. Warm-up of choice

2. Exercises
    a. Ankle Circles: 1 set of 10 rotations clockwise and counter-clockwise for each ankle.
    b. Neck Flexion: 1 set of 8 reps
    c. Seated Cat-Cow: 1 set of 8 reps
    d. Triceps Kickbacks: 1 set of 8 reps on each side
    e. Rowing Twists: 1 set of 8 reps to each side
3. Cooldown of choice

Tuesday

1. Warm-up of choice
2. Exercises
    a. Hip Marching: 1 set of 1-minute marching
    b. Neck Rotations: 1 set of 6 reps on each side
    c. Gentle Twist: 1 set of 6 reps on each side
    d. Elbow Side Extensions: 1 set of 8 reps
    e. Jumping Jacks: 1 set of 10 reps
3. Cooldown of choice

Wednesday

1. Warm-up of choice
2. Exercises
    a. Leg and Hip Extension: 1 set of 8 reps for each leg
    b. Levator Scapular: 1 set of 20-second hold
    c. Lumbar Extension: 1 set of 5 deep breath hold
    d. Tricep Lifts: 1 set of 8 reps
    e. Bicycle: 1 set of 6 reps of forward and backward rotations on each side
3. Cooldown of choice

Thursday

1. Warm-up of choice
2. Exercise
    a. Seated Hip and Knee Extension: 1 set of 6 reps for each leg
    b. Shoulder Rolls: 1 set of 8 reps
    c. Lumbar Side Flexion: 1 set of 8 reps for each side
    d. Bicep curls: 1 set of 8 reps for each side
    e. Hip flexors: 1 set of 20-second hold on each side

3. Cooldown of choice

Friday

1. Warm-up of choice
2. Exercise
   a. Standing Knee Flexion: 1 set of 8 reps for each leg
   b. Bicep Curl Into Shoulder Press: 1 set of 8 reps
   c. Seated Roll Down: 1 set of 6 reps
   d. Overhead Tricep Extension: 1 set of 8 reps for each side
   e. Flutter Kicks: 1 set of 30-second kicks
3. Cooldown of choice

Saturday

1. Warm-up of choice
2. Exercise
   a. Ankle pumps: 1 set of 8 reps up and down.
   b. Shoulder Flexions: 1 set of 8 reps
   c. Thoracic Rotation: 1 set of 6 reps for each side
   d. Wrist Flexion and Extension: 1 set of 8 reps for each side
   e. Seated Half Rollbacks: 1 set of 8 reps

3. Cooldown of choice

Sunday

1. Warm-up of choice
2. Exercise
   a. Calf Raises: 1 set of 8 reps.
   b. Shoulder Circles: 1 set of 8 reps forward and back rotation
   c. 90° Lateral Stretch: 1 set of 15-second hold
   d. Squeeze: 1 set of 8 reps for each side
   e. Leg Taps: 1 set of 8 reps
3. Cooldown of choice

Six-Day Targeted Workout Program

Targeted workouts focus on one body section that we want to improve. Instead of performing all seven exercises in that body section, we select a few that we want to concentrate on and add more sets. Alternatively, we utilize specific warm-ups for core, ankle, and legs. Change which exercises you do for each body section when you feel you have made the progress you want.

Monday: Ankle and Leg

1. Ankle and Leg Warm-up
2. Exercise

   a. Hip marching: 2 sets of 8 reps on each leg with 90 seconds of rest between sets

   b. Standing hip extension: 2 sets of 8 reps with 90 seconds of rest between sets

   c. Calf raises: 2 sets of 8 reps with 90 seconds of rest between sets

3. Cooldown of choice

Tuesday: Neck and Shoulders

1. Warm-up of choice

2. Exercise

   a. Bicep Curl Into Shoulder Press: 2 sets of 8 reps with 90 seconds of rest between sets

   b. Shoulder Flexions: 2 sets of 8 reps with 90 seconds of rest between sets

   c. Shoulder Circles: 2 sets of 8 reps with 90 seconds of rest between sets

3. Cooldown of choice

Wednesday: Core

1. Core Warm-up

   a. Bicycle: 2 sets of 6 reps of forward and backward rotations on each leg with 90 seconds of rest between sets

b. Leg taps: 2 sets of 8 reps with 90 seconds of rest between sets

c. Flutter kicks: 2 sets of 30 seconds with 90 seconds of rest between sets

2. Cooldown

Thursday: Upper and Lower Back

1. Warm-up of choice
2. Exercise

   a. Seated Cat-Cow: 2 sets of 8 reps with 90 seconds of rest between sets

   b. Lumbar Side Flexion: 2 sets of 6 reps on both sides with 90 seconds of rest between sets

   c. Thoracic Rotation: 2 sets of 6 reps on both sides with 90 seconds of rest between sets

3. Cooldown of choice

Friday: Arm, Wrist and Hand

1. Warm-up of choice
2. Exercise

   a. Tricep Kickbacks: 2 sets of 8 reps for each arm with 90 seconds of rest between sets

   b. Tricep Lifts: 2 sets of 8 reps with 90 seconds of rest between sets

   c. Squeeze: 2 sets of 8 reps for each hand with 90 seconds of rest between sets

3. Cooldown of choice

Saturday: Core

1. Core Warm-up
2. Exercise
   a. Bicycle: 2 sets of 6 reps of forward and backward rotations on each leg with 90 seconds of rest between sets
   b. Leg taps: 2 sets of 8 reps with 90 seconds of rest between sets
   c. Flutter kicks: 2 sets of 30 seconds with 90 seconds of rest between sets
3. Cooldown of choice

Sunday: Rest day

1. Take a day to rest.

Like that, you have a whole plan and base for your routines that can adapt to meet yourself where you are. Feel free to tweak your schedule, reduce or increase your sets or reps and modify the exercises to your needs. You are taking extraordinary steps to improve your physical wellness, allowing you to enjoy all aspects of your life.

Incorporating Chair Exercises Into Your Daily Routine

Whether you are new to exercise, coming back from a long period of rest, or are a seasoned pro, there are times when our routines get out of flow, and we need gentle reminders to get back into things.

Below are some gentle reminders, proven habits, tips, and tricks that steer us back toward our goals.

Keep Your Sessions Short and Sweet

An all-or-nothing mindset is one of my pet peeves regarding fitness and health. We become conditioned to believe that we must give it everything we have all the time to see results or benefit from our efforts.

You do not have to push yourself hard, especially in the beginning. You don't have an hour during your day to exercise? That's fine—you can shorten your session or break it up throughout the day. According to Miller (n.d.), research has shown that multiple bursts of exercise performed at intervals throughout the day significantly benefit our health.

Look for small ways to build exercise into your routine. If you take a quick break at a desk, why not choose an easy chair warm-up and stretch routine? These can be short five-minute breaks that not only add up to your daily exercise amount but can also give you a lovely mental break from work.

Ease Into Things

We have mentioned this before, but it is an important aspect of all fitness endeavors to gradually build up to an intensity and activity level you feel comfortable with and allows you to progress.

We never want to force anything, potentially leading to burnout or injury. Slow and steady progress is still progress.

Permit Yourself to Grow

It may be easy to compare yourself and your fitness levels to others, or perhaps you have the habit of comparing yourself to the younger version of yourself; however, we are in a different chapter of our lives, and our capabilities are different. The exercises can be adapted and tailored to where you are now and scaled to where you want to be. It is excellent because our needs are also different during this stage of our lives, and our workout routine should reflect that and change and adapt as we do.

Schedule Your Workouts

Think of it as booking a meeting or taking yourself on a date.

Commit to a manageable schedule for a few weeks to help you build a habit. Once established, it will be easier for you to work towards your goals.

Miller (n.d.) recommends that you exercise early in the morning. It gets it done and out of the way, allowing you to focus on the rest of your day's activities. If you can manage it, do your exercises early and tick it off your to-do list.

Keep It Fresh and Exciting

The key to maintaining a good workout routine is to keep it exciting. Doing the same exercises week after week will cause boredom unless we improve and add additional elements. Riding on the initial enthusiasm is easy, but we must continue fueling that drive. You can rotate which exercises you do in each workout, tempos, resistances, and even place your chair in a different location. Variety will keep things fresh and exciting, so factor it in as you plan your routine.

Make Exercise a Part of Your Identity

It can be disheartening when you give reasons for exercising that are usually negative and based on dreary potential outcomes of aging. You may fall, you may lose independence, or you may become sick. Instead, I want us to think of the positive results of exercising and what that means for us.

Instead of being people afraid of aging and losing our abilities and independence, we are embracing the changes. We are healthy individuals who know how to look after ourselves and prioritize our well-being. We are aging gracefully and will continue to be strong and capable in all areas of our lives.

Record Your Progress

Write down how your workouts went, how many repetitions you performed, and the sets. Record how you felt afterward to see how your body reacts to your training. Reviewing your experiences will help you know when is the right time to take the next step in progressive overload. If your journal consistently shows you're breezing through your exercises, feeling little to no resistance or fatigue, it might be time to dial things up a notch. But don't rush; let your journal be a testament to your journey, reminding you of your starting point and the strides you've made.

Additionally, looking back at your records can provide a motivational boost when you feel like you're not progressing. You might be surprised by how far you've come over weeks or months. It's also an excellent tool for self-reflection. If you find a particular exercise consistently leaves you feeling drained or causes discomfort, it's an indication to revisit your form or consider if it aligns with your goals and physical capacity.

Be Your Own Hype Person

Lasting, meaningful progress takes time, especially regarding health and wellness. Although all small changes count, it can sometimes be frustrating when we need to wait in order to see the results of our growth.

Always celebrate your small wins, no matter how inconsequential they might be. Small wins keep you motivated and confident when your long-term goals grow to fruition.

Reward Yourself

Remember those small milestones? Celebrate them and reward yourself when you accomplish them.

I usually reward myself with something fitness-related, but you should choose something that resonates with you and appropriately celebrates your achievements.

Hold Yourself Accountable

I have a workout buddy. I text them or call them once I have done my chair exercises for the day, and we chat about my progress, subsequent goals, and especially my struggles.

It is important to have someone you can share your journey with, such as your family, friends, and neighbors. Let them know your goals, ask them to check on you, and follow your progress.

Revisit Your Goals Often

Goals guide our fitness journey, but the underlying motivation – our "why" – gives them true power. It's not just about the dream but its deeper purpose.

At times, the exercise routine can make us lose sight of our progress or even the initial reasons we began. Regularly reflecting upon our achievements and the reasons behind our aspirations can reignite our drive and help us adapt our goals as we evolve.

For instance, I once aimed to stand on one leg for a minute on each side without support. While it might seem like a simple objective, I delved deeper to uncover its significance. Asking myself "why" repeatedly revealed a profound motivation:

> Why balance on one leg?
> Because it signifies my capability.
> And why is that essential?
> It means I can perform daily tasks with ease.
> And its importance?
> So I can confidently engage in activities with my grandchildren.

This realization reshaped my perspective. My objective wasn't just about balance but cherishing active moments with loved ones. Such insights can dramatically amplify motivation.

As you proceed, I encourage you to introspect on your goals regularly. Dive deep to uncover your true "why" and let it guide and energize your journey. Document these reflections and return to them, ensuring they remain at the heart of your endeavors.

Crafting a routine is like laying the foundation for a house. It provides stability, direction, and a sense of purpose to our fitness journey. As each week unfolds and you navigate through your routines, remember that every step, every exercise, and every moment of dedication is a brick you're adding to the tower of your health and well-being. This journey is uniquely yours, and this chapter has been about providing you with the tools and guidance to make it truly remarkable. Embrace the week ahead, stay committed to your routine, and, most importantly, cherish each new day's progress and growth.

Sharing Your Wisdom

With every exercise and insight you've gained from this book, it's now an opportunity to share the gift of mobility and well-being with others on the same journey.

Simply by leaving your genuine and honest review of this book on Amazon, you guide other seniors and their families toward a brighter, more active, and more fulfilling path in their golden years. Your insights will point them to the transformative power of these chair exercises and the potential for rejuvenated spirit and passion.

Thank you for your contribution. The journey to graceful aging is made richer when we share our experiences – and you're playing an essential role in enlightening that path for many.

Scan the QR code below

Conclusion

It feels good to be strong. Life is much more fulfilling and easier to navigate when we can trust our bodies to do what we need when we need it to. We eliminate fear. We keep our bravery, curiosity, and willingness to continue exploring the world. We should never have to give that up.

Society often frames aging as a journey towards diminished competence and independence, which can lead to unnecessary stress and fear. It suggests we'll face physical limitations, mental decline, and become ever-reliant on our loved ones or nursing homes. However, it's essential to remember that aging is a natural and beautiful part of life. Instead of succumbing to societal pressures and fearing the inevitable passage of time, we should embrace the wisdom, experience, and growth that come with each passing year. Every moment spent worrying about aging is a moment less spent on living. Let's choose to live fully, celebrating every stage of life's remarkable journey.

I am very passionate about chair exercises and exercise in general. A simple change to your lifestyle, such as the introduction of exercise, can make a world of difference to your lifestyle. We know the benefits of exercise. We need to nudge ourselves into action, and this is my nudge for you.

We deserve many years of joy, vitality, independence, and comfort. Let's change what it means to get older. Let's take our health, well-being, and future into our own hands. You have all the tools that you need. You do not need to spend large amounts of money on gym fees, coaches, or fitness classes—all you need is this book and your favorite chair to start.

Remember Harriet? She didn't let age slow her down, and exercise fueled that fire. I didn't mention before that Harriet's vitality and exuberance were not always there, and she had a period in life just before entering the assisted living facility where she developed depression. She had resigned herself to believe she was getting older and that her best years were behind her. She lost her spark and zeal.

At the insistence of her daughter, she took some group exercise classes. She was suddenly surrounded by people of all ages with different fitness levels. She began to lay a foundation of health for herself, which she took with her as she moved into the assisted living facility. Harriet continues her daily chair exercise routine and has recruited others to join her. Between them all, they love both the daily challenge and that they are breaking the preconceived notions of what it means to get older. Harriet was a beacon of inspiration for me when I first met her and saw how she still went through life, ignoring (and breaking) all the stigmas around getting older. She is the same for her fellow housemates.

She is not only an agile, strong, and physically capable inspiration to us all, but she has shown us how exercise can help you take control of your mental health. Her confidence, fearlessness, and positivity provide a beacon of hopefulness and belief in our continued chances to reach our potential.

So Harriet's story is not just about muscle, weight loss, exercise, and health: It is a story of the human spirit, which we should never let waiver. Her story is about rising above any challenges, whether it's in our control or not. It is about redefining what it means to age gracefully and a reminder that dreams or goals have no expiration date. Instead, aging opens up a whole new world of opportunities and strength.

So as this book comes to a close, I remind you that no matter where you are in your journey, you always have the option to start anew, to push your boundaries, and to discover your strength. Age is just a number. There are no limits to our potential.

So embrace each possibility that comes with each new year, and find your own "Harriet" within yourself. Here is to your future filled with ongoing opportunities and the joy of embracing life at every stage.

Continuing your workout routine, building and maintaining strength, mobility, flexibility, and balance for all body parts. You can significantly improve the quality of your life and autonomy, especially in later years. Whether it's reaching for an item on a high shelf or stabilizing oneself after a misstep, every exercise plays a part in holistic health, well-being, and independence.

Glossary

Chronic illness: A disease lasting more than three months is considered a chronic illness.

Extension: A movement that increases the angle between two body parts, such as straightening the elbow, which moves the forearm away from the upper arm,

Flexion: A movement that decreases the angle between two body parts, such as bending the elbow, which brings the forearm closer to the upper arm.

Physical therapy: The practice of using physical activities to treat injuries or diseases.

Proprioception: The body's ability to sense its position and movement in space.

Quality of life: Your well-being and how fulfilling your life is. Quality of life refers to emotional, spiritual, and physical well-being.

Optional Amazon Purchases

Please note that we suggest products on Amazon.com, based on our prior purchases and comprehensive research into product quality and customer reviews. We recommend items that we believe are high-quality products. However, we do not receive any form of royalties or commissions for these recommendations. These products are provided solely for your convenience and information. We encourage users to carry out their own due diligence to ensure that the product is the right size, weight, or fit for their individual needs before making a purchase. While we have made efforts to suggest reliable products, the decision to purchase remains your own. Any issues with a product, including, but not limited to, dissatisfaction with the quality, condition, or overall performance of the product, are the sole responsibility of the purchaser. We are not liable for any purchase decisions or for any issues arising out of the use of these products.

Products

Simply type these items into Amazon's search engine.

- Amazon Basics Neoprene Workout Dumbbell - Qty (2) 2lbs, Qty (2) 3lbs & Qty (2) 5lbs, total (6) dumbbells
- Starktape Resistance Bands. **100% Malaysian Natural Latex Band**. Perfect for Physical Therapy, Home Exercise, Yoga, Pilates, Gym, Rehab Training. No Scent, No Powder

- Starktape Resistance Bands Set. 5 Pack **Non-Latex** Physical Therapy, Professional Elastic Band. Perfect for Home Exercise, Workout, Strength Training, Yoga, Pilates, Rehab or Gym Leg Upper, Lower Body
- GOZATO 5-Pack Hand Exercise Balls - Physical & Occupational Therapy Kit for Strengthening Grip & Reducing Stiffness - Arthritis Pain Relief Exerciser for Physical Therapy, Fidget, Stress Relief
- VINSGUIR Workout Gloves for Men and Women, Weight Lifting Gloves with Excellent Grip, Lightweight Gym Gloves for Weightlifting, Cycling, Exercise, Training, Pull ups, Fitness, Climbing and Rowing

References

-Alverson, M. (2021, October 10). *Unlock the benefits of neck training: Improve your posture, increase strength, and reduce injury risk.* The Rack. https://therackapc.com/reasons-why-you-should-train-the-neck/

-American Psychological Association. (2021, September). *Older adults' health and age-related changes.* Apa.org. https://www.apa.org/pi/aging/resources/guides/older

-Baylor University. (2019, November 6). *Mobility loss puts older adults at risk: Research shows exercise can help | online graduate programs | Baylor.* BAY-UMT. https://onlinegrad.baylor.edu/resources/mobility-exercises/

-Bedosky, L. (2021, March 13). *The best core exercises for seniors.* Get Healthy U. https://gethealthyu.com/best-core-exercises-for-seniors/

-Best Health. (2000, January 1). *Prayer stretch.* Best Health. https://www.besthealthmag.ca/article/prayer-stretch/

-Better Health Channel. (2012). *Physical activity – setting yourself goals.* Vic.gov.au. https://www.betterhealth.vic.gov.au/health/healthyliving/physical-activity-setting-yourself-goals

-Biddulph, M. (2022, November 4). *How to use resistance bands: A guide for beginners.* Livescienc e.com. https://www.livescience.com/how-to-use-resistance-bands

-Blog, I. (2021, April 14). *7 exercise safety tips for seniors.* Immaculate Home Care. https://immaculatehcs.com/blog/7-exercise-safety-tips-for-seniors/

-Better Health Channel. (2015). *Exercise safety.* Vic.gov.au. https://www.betterhealth.vic.gov.au/health/healthyliving/exercise-safety%23exercise-safety-advice

-*Betty Friedan quotes.* (n.d.). BrainyQuote.com. https://www.brainyquote.com/quotes/betty_friedan_383994

-Blue Zones. (2015). *History of Blue Zones - Blue Zones.* Blue Zones. https://www.bluezones.com/about/history/

-Care Link. (2021, September 21). *Benefits of chair exercises for seniors.* CareLink. https://www.carelink.org/benefits-of-chair-exercises-for-seniors/

-CDC. (2019). *How much physical activity do older adults need?* Centers for Disease Control and Prevention. https://www.cdc.gov/physicalactivity/basics/older_adults/index.htm

-CDC. (2020, July 6). *Keep on your feet.* Centers for Disease Control and Prevention.

https://www.cdc.gov/injury/features/older-adult-falls/
-Cerqua, P. (2022, May 4). *6 ways to motivate yourself to work out.* WikiHow. https://www.wiki-how.com/Motivate-Yourself-to-Work-Out
-Chertoff, J. (2020, July 30). *Progressive overload: What it is, examples, and tips.* Healthline. https://www.healthline.com/health/progressive-overload#ways-to-do-it
-Cyprus, S. (2023, April 26). *What are chair exercises?* Wise-geek.com
. https://www.wise-geek.com/what-are-chair-exercises.htm
-Dagnino, A. P. A., & Campos, M. M. (2022). *Chronic pain in the elderly: Mechanisms and perspectives.* Frontiers in Human Neuroscience, *16.* https://doi.org/10.3389/fnhum.2022.736688
-Elder Gym. (n.d.). *Shoulder muscle workout for seniors and the elderly* . Eldergym.com. https://el-dergym.com/shoulder-muscle-workout/
-Excellence in Fitness. (n.d.). *Top 10 benefits seniors experience when exercising*. Excellence in Fitness. https://www.excellenceinfitness.com/blog/benefits-exercising-seniors
-Fancy, L. (2020, March 20). *6 ways for seniors to stay safe while exercising.* Home Care Assistance Winnipeg, Manitoba. https://www.homecareassistancewinnipeg.ca/how-can-ag-ing-adults-exercise-safely/
-Fiorito, R. (2017, February 17). *De-stress instantly with this easy chair yoga flow.* PureWow. https://www.purewow.com/wellness/chair-yoga-poses
-Freiberger, E., Sieber, C. C., & Kob, R. (2020). *Mobility in older community-dwelling persons: A narrative review.* Frontiers in Physiology, *11.* https://doi.org/10.3389/fphys.2020.00881
-Gilson, J. (2018, September 12). *How to create your own workout plan: A guide for beginners.* Whole Life Challenge. https://www.wholelifechallenge.com/how-to-design-your-own-work-out-program-a-guide-for-beginners/
-Hanna, S., & Norman, A. (n.d.). *Chair-based exercise.* South Cambridgeshire Falls Pre-vention Service. https://laterlifetraining.co.uk/wp-content/uploads/2011/01/Chair-Based-Exer-cise_Cambridge.pdf
-Heather. (2022, August 15). 17 ways to stay motivated to exercise. Better Living. https://onbet-terliving.com/fitness-motivation/
-*Jackie Joyner-Kersee quotes.* (n.d.). BrainyQuote.com
. https://www.brainyquote.com/quotes/jackie_joynerkersee_126146
-*Jillian Michaels quotes* . (n.d.). Goodreads.com. https://www.goodreads.com/au-thor/quotes/5106.Jillian_Michaels%23
-*John F. Kennedy quotes.* (n.d.). BrainyQuote.com
. https://www.brainyquote.com/quotes/john_f_kennedy_131489-
-John Hopkins Medicine. (n.d.). *Osteoporosis: What you need to know as you age.* Hopkinsmedicine.org. Retrieved May 10, 2023, from https://www.hopkinsmedicine.org/health/conditions-and-diseases/osteoporosis/osteo-porosis-what-you-need-to-know-as—you-age#:~:text=From%20about%20age%2025%20to
-Kutcher, M. (n.d.). *Best seated warm up routine for seniors | More Life Health.* More Life Health -

Seniors Health & Fitness. Retrieved May 21, 2023, from https://morelifehealth.com/articles/seated-warmup-routine
-Kutcher, M. (n.d.-a). *Exercise library for seniors.* More Life Health - Seniors Health & Fitness. Retrieved May 28, 2023, from https://morelifehealth.com/exercise-library
-Kutcher, M. (n.d.-b). *Knee flexion exercise technique for seniors | More Life Health.* More Life Health - Seniors Health & Fitness. Retrieved May 27, 2023, from https://morelifehealth.com/knee-flexions
-Kutcher, M. (n.d.-c). *Shoulder roll exercise technique for seniors | More Life Health.* More Life Health - Seniors Health & Fitness. Retrieved May 28, 2023, from https://morelifehealth.com/shoulder-rolls
-Kutcher, M. (n.d.-d). *Seated hip flexions exercise for seniors | More Life Health.* More Life Health - Seniors Health & Fitness. Retrieved May 27, 2023, from https://morelifehealth.com/seated-hip-flexions
-Kutcher, M. (2018, November 7). *Neck exercises for seniors | simple neck stretches for seniors | More Life Health* [Video]. Youtube. https://www.youtube.com/watch?v=r0c_5gZ2Z2k
-Kutcher, M. (2019a, April 10). *Best arms, shoulders & legs exercises for seniors! | seniors' chair exercises | More Life Health* [Video]. YouTube. https://www.youtube.com/watch?v=NHwWx2OhRMs
-Kutcher, M. (2019, July 3). *Best neck exercises for seniors | seniors posture & mobility.* More Life Health - Seniors Health & Fitness. https://morelifehealth.com/articles/best-neck-exercises-for-seniors
-Kutcher, M. (2020, April 19). *Simple seated core workout for seniors (10-minutes) | More Life Health* [Video]. YouTube. https://www.youtube.com/watch?v=DsH3dafrlsc
-Living Maples. (2021, January 23). *Best exercise shoes for seniors: Comfort in every step.* Living Maples. https://livingmaples.com/mag/best-exercise-shoes-for-seniors/
-Lo'Aids. (2021, April 26). *50 inspiring senior fitness quotes to keep you moving.*
-Loaids.com. https://loaids.com/senior-fitness-quotes/
-MacDonald, J. (n.d.). *Train with Joan.* Mysite. https://www.trainwithjoanofficial.com/
-May, K. (2020, March 27). *6 conditions that lead to mobility limitations in seniors.* Home Care Assistance of Amarillo, TX. https://www.homecareassistanceamarillo.com/what-can-cause-my-elderly-parent-to-have-reduced-mobility/
-Mayo Clinic. (2020, November 19). Aging: What to expect. Mayo Clinic. https://www.mayoclinic.org/healthy-lifestyle/healthy-aging/in-depth/aging/art-20046070
-McCoy, J. (2018). *11 tips to set realistic fitness goals you'll actually achieve, according to top trainers.* SELF. https://www.self.com/story/how-to-set-realistic-fitness-goals
-Melone, L. (n.d.). *7 dynamic warm ups.* Arthritis.org. https://www.arthritis.org/health-wellness/healthy-living/physical-activity/other-activities/7-dynamic-warm-ups
-Miller, B. (n.d.). *7 tips for making exercise part of your daily routine.* Happify.com . https://www.happify.com/hd/7-tips-for-making-exercise-part-of-your-daily-routine/
-mmLearn.org. (n.d.). *Nine Benefits of Yoga for Seniors.* Training.mmlearn.org. https://train-

ing.mmlearn.org/blog/nine-benefits-of-yoga-for-seniors
-More Life Health. (2019, April 1). *Standing warm-up routine for seniors (do before undertaking exercise) | more life health* [Video]. YouTube. https://www.youtube.com/watch?v=b2DYU7ZQgN0
-More Life Health. (2021, January 31). **NEW* SEATED warm up for seniors | More Life Health* [Video]. YouTube. https://www.youtube.com/watch?v=MljaW8zv5bg
-Moyer, C. (2020, September 23). *How aging affects your feet.* Verywell Health. https://www.verywellhealth.com/how-aging-affects-your-feet-1337806
-Muscleblaze. (n.d.). *Benefits of a warm up before a workout.* Muscleblaze. https://www.muscleblaze.com/articles/Exercise/benefits-of-a-warm-up-before-a-workout/4598
-National Council of Aging. (n.d.). *The life-changing benefits of exercise after 60.* Ncoa.org. Retrieved May 10, 2023, from https://ncoa.org/article/the-life-changing-benefits-of-exercise-after-60
-National Council On Aging. (2023, March 13). *Get the facts on falls prevention.* Ncoa.org. https://ncoa.org/article/get-the-facts-on-falls-prevention
-National Institute on Aging. (2020, April 3). *How older adults can get started with exercise.* National Institute on Aging. https://www.nia.nih.gov/health/how-older-adults-can-get-started-exercise
-Nera, S. (2021, March 8). *Exercise safety tips for seniors and older adults: Preventing injury.* Hello Doctor. https://hellodoctor.com.ph/healthy-aging/exercise-safety-tips-for-seniors/
-NHS. (2022, January 26). *Sitting exercises.* Nhs.uk. https://www.nhs.uk/live-well/exercise/strength-and-flexibility-exercises/sitting-exercises/
-Pahla B, Weight Loss Coach for Women Over 50. (2019, April 12). *Energizing seated stretch | warm up, cool down or desk break workout | 5 minute friday fix* [Video]. YouTube. https://www.youtube.com/watch?v=SCoYPfYJPyI&t=32s
-Peterson, J. A. (2009). *10 common-sense safety tips for exercise enthusiasts.* ACSM's Health & Fitness Journal, *13*(2), 46. https://doi.org/10.1249/fit.0b013e3181998c64
-Pike, J. M., Singh, S. K., Barfield, W. R., Schoch, B., Friedman, R. J., & Eichinger, J. K. (2022). *Impact of age on shoulder range of motion and strength.* JSES International, *6*(6), 1029–1033. https://doi.org/10.1016/j.jseint.2022.08.016
-Precision Nutrition. (2019). *Worksheet: The 5 whys for clients.* https://assets.precisionnutrition.com/2019/08/worksheet-the-5-whys.pdf
-Provectus Physiotherapy & Health Services. (2022, September 1). *Progressive overload for seniors.* Provectus - Home Physiotherapy in Vancouver. https://provectusphysiotherapy.ca/senior-care
-*A quote by Bill Loguidice.* (n.d.). Goodreads.com
. https://www.goodreads.com/quotes/514661-it-s-easier-to-stay-in-shape-if-you-never-let
-Reinhardt Chiropractic. (2017, January 1). *5 stretches to sooth neck pain.* Reinhardt Chiropractic. https://www.reinhardtchiropractic.com/blog/5-stretches-for-neck-pain/
-Restorative Strength. (n.d.). *Recovering from injury faster in seniors.* Restorativestrength.com. Retrieved June 3, 2023, from https://restorativestrength.com/recovering-from-injury-in-seniors/

-Robeck, I. (2012). *Chronic pain in the elderly: Special challenges.* Practical Pain Management. https://www.practicalpainmanagement.com/pain/chronic-pain-elderly-special-challenges
-Robinson, L. (2019). *Senior exercise and fitness tips.* HelpGuide.org
. https://www.helpguide.org/articles/healthy-living/exercise-and-fitness-as-you-age.htm
-Scalena, M. (2021, May 19). *7 benefits of daily seated exercise.* Sunshine Centres for Seniors. https://sunshinecentres.com/7-benefits-of-daily-seated-exercise/
-Schrift , D. (n.d.). *Upper back stretches for seniors.* Eldergym.com. https://eldergym.com/upper-back-stretches-for-seniors/
-Shah, M. (2022, March 11). *You are never too old to set another goal or to dream a new dream.* SetQuotes. https://www.setquotes.com/you-are-never-too-old-to-set-another-goal-or-dream/
-Sofia, C. (2019, March 25). *5 seated chair exercises for back pain.* Coach Sofia Fitness. https://www.coachsofiafitness.com/chair-exercises-and-stretches-for-back-pain-and-stiffness/
-SonderCare. (n.d.). *What are common mobility Issues in old age?.* Sondercare.com. Retrieved May 3, 2023, from https://www.sondercare.com/learn/mobility-disability/what-common-mobility-issues-old-age/
-Spring Hills. (2020, January 28). *How exercise can help you recover from injuries and illness.* Spring Hills | Senior Communities. https://www.springhills.com/resources/how-exercise-can-help-you-recover-from-injuries-and-illness/
-Stelter, G. (2014, August 14). *5 seated back pain stretches for seniors.* Healthline. https://www.healthline.com/health/back-pain/stretches-for-seniors#The%20takeaway
-Street Workout St Kilda. (2021, July 25). *Ankle pumps exercise - complete guide.* Streetworkoutst kilda.com. https://www.streetworkoutstkilda.com/ankle-pumps-exercise/
-Sweat. (2019, January 3). *How to set SMART fitness goals.* SWEAT. https://www.sweat.com/blogs/life/goal-setting
-*The most common causes of limited mobility in seniors.* (n.d.). Hdfcergo.com. Retrieved May 4, 2023, from https://www.hdfcergo.com/health-insurance/wellness-corner/common-causes-for-limited-mobility-in-seniors
-The U.S. Department of Health and Human Services. (n.d.). *Physical activity guidelines for Americans 2nd edition.* https://health.gov/sites/default/files/2019-09/Physical_Activity_Guidelines_2nd_edition.pdf#page=73
-Viggiano, M. (2019, February 14). *Returning to exercise after a fall.* AIM Human Performance. https://www.aimhumanperformance.com/blog/2019/2/14/returning-to-exercise-after-a-fall
-Vive Health. (2020, February 10). *Seated ankle rotation chair exercise* [Video]. YouTube. https://www.youtube.com/watch?v=sYAGbGEQMGE
-Weber, J. (2021, November 10). *Why is core strength exercise so important for seniors?* The Fitness Frame. https://thefitnessframe.com/seniors-core-strength-exercise
-Weil, A. (n.d.). Breathing exercises: 4-7-8 breath. DrWeil.com. Retrieved June 27, 2023, from

https://www.drweil.com/videos-features/videos/breathing-exercises-4-7-8-breath/
-Weil, R. (2022, May 2). *Senior exercise: It's never too late to start exercising.* MedicineNet. https://www.medicinenet.com/senior_exercise/article.htm
-Wilkins, B. (2022, June 9). *Gal Gadot and Kate Upton swear by progressive overload - here's what it is, and how to do it.* Women's Health. https://www.womenshealthmag.com/uk/fitness/workouts/a40218848/progressive-overload/
-*Wrist tendinitis: Exercises.* (n.d.). Myhealth.alberta.ca. https://myhealth.alberta.ca/Health/aftercareinformation/pages/conditions.aspx?hwid=bo1652
-Zorzan , N. (2022, October 31). *Best chair exercises for seniors: Safe and easy workouts.* Medicalnewstoday.com. https://www.medicalnewstoday.com/articles/chair-exercises-for-seniors#side-bend

Made in United States
Troutdale, OR
08/17/2024